The Most Precious Gift

Lawrence Liebling

Silent River Press

❖ ❖

First Printing 2000   First Edition 2000   ISBN9642872-0

Silent River Press
2971 Bellmore Avenue
Bellmore, New York 11710

Cover design using Corel Draw by:
Allen Burdowski, Lawrence Liebling and Jerry Seinfeld
Printed and bound in the United States of America.

Library of Congress Cataloging-in-Publication Data

Liebling, Lawrence, 1952-
   The most precious gift / Lawrence Liebling.—1ˢᵗ ed.
   p. cm.
   ISBN 0-9642874-2-0 (hardcover : alk. Paper)
      1. Liebling, Lawrence, 1952- 2. Kidneys—Transplantation—
         Patients—Biography. I. Title.

RD575 .L54 2000
362.1'974610592'092—dc21
[B]
                                                           99-054867

This book is dedicated with love

to

Carolyn and Josh

&

Mom, Dad and Debbie

Acknowledgments

❖

Creativity blooms with the encouragement and enthusiasm of others. It is with great pleasure that I thank the following people for sharing their thoughts and ideas with me.

I would like to express my sincere thanks to Elizabeth Clark, Robin Sherman, Jacki Kaplan, Nancy Geller, Karen Greene, Sam and Sherry Husney, Lynn and Sol Hesney, Steve Freeman, Charles Klein, and Norman Gertner. They are all dear friends who took time from their busy schedules to read The Most Precious Gift and share their reactions and personal feelings with me. I am forever thankful and appreciative of their efforts and their kindness.

A special acknowledgment to Dan Strone who prompted me to search my inner voice and give more of myself to this book after each draft. His vigilance is most appreciated.

I would like to express my thanks to Diane Schoenberg who skillfully copy edited this book. More than that, her warm friendship made it a pleasure to collaborate on this project.

To Allen and Susan Burdowski my deepest appreciation not only for their unceasing guidance and support, but also for their everlasting friendship. In addition, I want to thank Allen for the countless hours he spent and fabulous job he did on the design of the front cover.

Nothing in our lives affect who we are more significantly than our families. I am grateful and blessed to share life with mine. Thanks to Betty Seinfeld whose love and advice cheer me on in everything I do. Thanks to Jerry Seinfeld, who makes the world laugh, and whom I know as kind, generous, and supportive. His help on the design of the front cover was invaluable. A special thanks to Jessica Seinfeld whose kind and gentle heart has enriched all of us and whose enthusiasm for this project is especially appreciated. With never-ending love and eternal gratitude, thanks to my mom and dad, Ed and Seena Liebling, who gave me life and who continually nurture me with their love. How thankful I am to my wife, Carolyn, and son, Josh, for the joy and sweetness they bring to me every day. Their love inspires my life and is infused in every step I take.

The Most Precious Gift

❖　❖　❖　❖

Time goes by so fast. Day after day, week by week, month by month, year after year, until a whole lifetime is done—come and gone almost in an instant. Our moments are strung together holding limit less possibilities. The scene is set for us everyday. Like clockwork the sun rises, waiting for the dreams and hopes of millions to unfold. Like clockwork the sun sets at the conclusion of the day, offering each of us an opportunity to reflect on who we are, where we have been, and where we would like to be.

The day turns into evening and our nights are filled with sleep's journey to a different plane. It's where unanswered questions sometimes find resolution. Then, morning awaits us again.

Our moments, strung together, form a rich tapestry of experiences that adorn our soul's eternal heart. We weave this vivid mosaic into a colorful portrait that makes up our lives.

From the highest peaks to the lowest depths, we yearn to journey toward wholeness. Sometimes we are fractured beyond immediate repair and wholeness looks like a daunting task never to be realized. Sometimes we feel confused and lost, our equilibrium gone; we teeter on the brink of despair.

Yet other times, though, we can peer into eternity and realize that being alive is truly sublime. We feel our own greatness, knowing that we are more than what we appear. We feel ourselves to be shining stars that are evolving, hurling toward breathtaking splendor.

Life is a mysterious gift. Often we sojourn to the depths of creation only to rise and crown it.

The things that happen to us, that make us who we are, happen for a reason. The sum of our days is more than just folly. Our lives point us to a greater reality that, when taken as a whole, tell us how far we've reached and how much further we have to go.

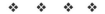

Part One:
The Morning of
September 1, 1996

❖ ❖ ❖ ❖

1

❖ ❖ ❖ ❖

The morning air gently comes streaming in through the half-open bedroom window. It's moist and pleasantly cool. Hovering between sleep and being awake, I find myself smiling, welcoming its embrace. As it washes over me, I rise through the final sequence of dreams and into wakefulness. But sleep feels so deliciously comforting; I can't quite rouse myself from its hold on me. I start to drift off again. Then my mind intrudes; I am awake and instantly struck by a sense of time. It starts to race through me and I feel its rhythm, moving forward.

It seems as though I slept through the night or at least I don't remember getting up, not even once. In contrast to the last several months which have been marked by many sleepless nights, I feel rested.

My wife, Carolyn, is still sleeping. Our dog, Molly, a golden retriever, stirs in the corner. I slip out of bed and automatically launch myself toward the bathroom and into the shower.

As the warm water soaks over me, I cover my eyes with my hands and start to cry. I can't stop. Just like yesterday and the day before. I try to take hold of myself, but I know it's of little use.

As quickly as it comes, the crying stops. Stepping out of the shower, I towel myself off, thankful that this wave of tears has subsided. I feel a sense of relief, but nothing is resolved.

As I emerge through the bathroom doorway, Molly is now propped up in her corner awaiting my arrival. Upon the sight of me, she wags her tail and smiles. I quickly and quietly get dressed. Carolyn loves her sleep and I do my best not to disturb her.

"Larry, why are you up so early?" She barely gets the garbled words out.

"It's all right, go back to…" but before I can finish, she's already gently breathing rhythmically and happily sleeping again, her dark brown hair falling peacefully against the pillow.

I'm drawn to the kitchen with thoughts of a cup of coffee and maybe some toast and jam. Walking out of the bedroom and down the hall, I pass Joshua's room. I look in on my son who has taken on his mother's love of sleep. In a few days, school will begin again and his lullaby summer mornings will be gone, replaced with the hectic schedule of an eighth grader.

I hear rustling coming from my bedroom. Molly turns the corner into the hallway, consenting to be an early morning companion. She almost always is.

We make our way down the hall and into the kitchen. The colors of the morning filter through the large kitchen windows, making their way from across the rooftops of the houses that line the street behind us. Soft golden threads fall across the flooring. The morning strikes my heart with its beauty, but it can't capture my soul. I am troubled by a melancholy that keeps me bound. Unresolved feeling. Everything that has happened to my sister seems so unsettled in my mind.

I briefly consider getting the morning newspaper lying in the driveway, but decide instead to forgo the day's headlines. Breakfast, too, has lost its appeal. "Molly, let's go sit in the back. We'll get some fresh air and clear our heads." She's eager to oblige and jumps down the stairs, prances through the den, and waits for me at the large sliding glass door that leads to the backyard.

Being careful not to disturb nature's work, I unlock the door and quietly glide it open. I feel the morning mist gently mingling with my breath. The air is crisp and laced with sweetness. The summer's sun continues to linger and its warmth filters through the coolness of the dawn.

The sunrise is a faithful reminder that life renews itself daily. Quiet and undisturbed, the morning is filled with sunlight that cascades silhouettes everywhere.

Molly takes off inspecting what she perceives as her backyard kingdom. The birds and squirrels are her subjects along with the trees and bushes.

Walking across the end of the brick patio, I take my place in a comfortable porch chair. Looking skyward, I breathe in the sunlight and think to myself, another morning, yet this morning seems different. It keeps enticing me to enjoy its beauty. More than that, it stirs feelings from a time long ago. Nature has always found a way to reach deep into my spirit.

It's hard to believe that it's been over twenty-two years. A lifetime away. So many things have happened. Yet that year and its consequences remain with me forever, reaching across time and space. And now, this very moment, its haunting echo floods my mind. Present events conspire to resurrect emotions long thought put to rest. They now surface as if to say, "It's time."

What happened then is directly connected to the tangled web of emotions I feel today. All that has transpired in between seems as if it were condensed into a single day. Yet, at the same time, so much has happened. So many moments to consider–times of joy and sorrow and despair and exhilaration.

The doorway of memory opens. Perhaps I stand at the threshold of a new understanding. Life seems to continually present new questions, as the old ones are resolved. It appears true understanding is an elusive prize, a fleeting moment, grasped, then gone.

Now questions of life and death and why some of us have to endure great hardship tug at my heart. Questions about my own life and how things have turned out are swirling around in my head.

That time twenty-two years ago comes crashing into the present. Who could deny how much it affected us? It was a time when life hung on the wings of angels. It would shape the way we would relate to each other for the rest of our lives.

My thoughts begin to roam. As easy as autumn leaves drift down a winding stream, I'm irresistibly drawn down river to thoughts long ago, to twenty-two years ago when as a young man of twenty-one, I was faced with a most unusual circumstance.

I remember it so well that my senses can conjure up the very scent, sight, and sound that surrounded it.

It was late January, a bitter-cold New York morning. Like today, the sun was shining boldly, but on that day its warmth was hardly a match for the bone-chilling freeze that blanketed the entire northeast region.

The traffic was heavy on the Clearview Expressway. I don't remember if it was due to roadwork, an accident, or just typical highway congestion. Whatever it was, a ride that usually takes an hour was now closing in on two. The fumes of the traffic easily passed through the car's exterior.

The four of us huddled in a blue Buick Riviera driving head-long to what was a defining moment for each of us. My mom and dad were sitting in the front seat and my sister, Debbie, and I were buckled in the back. All of us were wondering how the next days, weeks, and months were going to change our lives.

We were all pretty quiet. An occasional comment, or small talk, would disengage us from our separate thoughts. My dad anxiously wondered what was causing the holdup. "We should have been there an hour ago," he said as he loosened his grip on the side of the steering wheel and raised his open hand in mock disgust. My mom asked him to please drive with two hands and firmly insisted that we wouldn't get their any faster with his complaining.

My sister and I acknowledged their comments but were basically quiet, though I do recall trying to say something in an effort to make it seem like just another ordinary day. But, of course, it wasn't.

It wasn't because by tomorrow morning, my parents could lose one or both of their children. The flip side, though, was that if all went well, life could begin again. The grip of despair and fear that held their lives in limbo would be over.

As we finally arrived, my father drove up to the front entrance, dropped us off, and went to park the car. My mother told him, "Eddie, watch out for the ice on the walk back." "I'll be all right," he said. "Just take the kids in and I'll catch up."

The three of us got out of the car. My mom and sister got out of the passenger side and I slowly got out from the driver side. As I closed the door, I paused for a moment and felt as if I was leaving something behind. I walked over to where my mother and sister were waiting for me at the curb. We looked at each other for an instant, then walked together. As we stepped up to the front door, I thought to myself that I just wanted it to be over.

We quickly went in. There were lots of people, too many

people. The rushed atmosphere was a stark contrast to the solitude of the car ride. All the planning, the tests, the hopes, the dread, the waiting, and the anticipation were over. Not over in the sense that it was a conclusion, but over because the page was about to be turned in what seemed to be this never-ending saga. What was about to unfold was four years in the making. Everything that happened during the past few years was a prelude to this moment.

My mom walked us to the admitting office. "You're the Lieblings, aren't you? We've been expecting you. Please sit down." We reluctantly walked over to a series of dark wooden desks and chairs and quietly sat down. A tall woman with a kind face and a pleasing smile asked us who wanted to go first. Debbie and I looked at each other and shrugged our shoulders. Then, without hesitation, my Mom said, "Larry, let your sister go ahead of you." Without thinking twice, I said, "Okay." Debbie quickly gave her information.

Then it was my turn. The woman smiled at me and began to ask a few questions starting with my name, which I thought rather silly because she already knew who I was. She ran through the other questions quickly, then asked me to hold out my arm so she could put an ID bracelet around my wrist. I felt branded, marked for who knows what. Within a few minutes, we were both officially processed.

With that, the final stage was set in motion. The process was irreversible. I take that back. The process was irreversible the day my sister got sick. Her medical odyssey began when she was fourteen and, if you want to talk karma, probably the day she was born.

2

❖ ❖ ❖ ❖

"Larry?"

Suddenly, Carolyn jarred me from my trance back into the present.

"Larry, are you downstairs?"

"Yes."

"Is the dog with you?"

"Yeah, Molly and I are enjoying the morning air. Come down and join us."

Molly wags her tail, first slowly, then completely at the sound of my wife's voice. As Carolyn appears at the door, the dog races over to greet her.

"Good morning, Molly. What are you and Larry doing outside?"

"We got up early and didn't want to wake you and Josh so we thought it would be nice to sit outside."

"Did you have any breakfast yet?"

"I thought about a light bite, but Molly and I decided to come out here instead."

"I can see why, it's a beautiful morning. I can't remember the last time the air was crystal clear."

"Can you believe that the summer is over?

"I know, I feel the same way. With everything that happened over the last few months, it feels like summer completely passed us by."

"Before you turn around, it will be winter and we'll be digging ourselves out of the snow."

"And Josh will have his ears glued to the radio to see if school is closed."

Carolyn and I smiled at the thought.

"How did you sleep?" she asked.

"Okay I guess. How about you?"

"I was up in the middle of the night thinking about your sister."

"I know. I was just recalling the day we went into the hospital twenty-two years ago."

"My God! Is it that long ago?"

"I know it's hard to believe but it is."

"Do you want to talk about it?"

"I don't know what good it would do."

"Larry, if you talk things out, you'll feel much better."

"Maybe later. Right now, I just want to sit here for a while and try to sort it out in my own mind."

"All right, but remember I'm here if you need me."

With that, Carolyn hugged me around the neck and placed a soft kiss on the side of my head. I smiled and appreciatively kissed her cheek.

"Well, I'll go upstairs, take a shower, and get dressed. I'll see you two in a bit."

Carolyn disappeared beyond the sliding glass door and went

back upstairs. Molly stayed with me, curling herself by my feet. It was quiet again. All that caught my mind was the sound of my own breath. I closed my eyes and felt the warm morning sun streaming across my face. It kindled a longing for memories past. Once more I found myself thinking about Debbie again. I was only seventeen when she got sick, just out of high school and on the way to my first year of college.

For my entire life, my parents had nurtured me and given me the benefit of their life's experience. They instilled in me a sense of responsibility and taught me to be caring and respectful of others. Living in New York, Florida seemed like a long way off but I felt that it was time to fly away from the comfort of living with my family. Along with my sister, I had grown up in a relatively sheltered environment. Like many of their contemporaries, my parents settled in the newly-developed suburban communities outside of New York City.

It was a time of climbing shade trees in the backyard, going to drive-in movies on hot summer evenings, playing stickball in the schoolyard on a June day, and enjoying sleigh rides in the park during the winter's snowy months. Weekends included mowing the lawn in the summer and raking the leaves in the fall. When someone bought a new car, the whole block came out for a ride and shared in the spectacle. A shiny new car brought out all the "oohs" and "ahs." Every father had to then go home and explain to the rest of his family why a brand new Ford or Chevy wasn't going to be sitting in their driveway anytime soon.

My father commuted to New York City where he and my grandfather participated in the American dream of owning a small business. My dad worked hard, which included many late hours. Often he would be long gone by the time Debbie and I had to get up for school. Sometimes I'd hear the front door close, run into

21

my parents' room, and jump into his empty bed and cuddle within the warmth he left behind.

My mother encouraged him to be home on time for dinner so that, as a family, we would have an opportunity to be together and talk about what had happened to us during the day. Every night my mom would come in and tuck Debbie and me into our beds with heartening words and a tender hug. We shared in each other's lives and we were sustained and strengthened by a strong family identity.

From a very young age, I felt a responsibility for my little sister. Whenever I went out to play with the neighborhood kids, Debbie was always at my heels. Whether it was a game of football or riding bikes, she always insisted that she be included. Whatever I did or had, she wanted.

Sometimes a bunch of my friends would spend the afternoon at my house using clothespins to attach baseball cards to the spokes of our bikes. Debbie wasn't content just to watch. The motorized tapping sound the cards made wasn't about to be the private domain of my friends and me. Debbie insisted on joining the contest to produce the loudest and most elaborate card display. At my mom's insistence, I was to instruct her on the fine art of baseball-card powered cycling.

When we were small, my sister looked up to me. When I decided to take piano lessons, to the astonishment of no one, Debbie eagerly followed my lead. If I got to sit in the front seat of the car, Debbie wanted to sit in the front too. Soon, however, my sister realized she didn't have to do whatever I did. She found her own way, asserted her independence, and I was out as a guiding light.

Then, instead of emulating me, she competed with me. If I wanted to go to the movies, she wanted to go bowling. If my parents were taking us out to dinner and I wanted Italian food, she would want Chinese. We even disagreed over who had the fewest freckles–both of us considered them more than a minor annoyance. As most siblings do, we competed for our parents' attention.

Our roles developed differently. I was the older brother, responsible, and permitted certain things that she wasn't–like staying up later. She was the younger child, the baby, and she got the benefits of the trail I already blazed. She ended up getting away with things that I was denied at her age. I didn't feel any great despair when she got into trouble, which, of course, seemed less often then I did. And if I was caught at some undesirable deed, she took particular glee in seeing me banished to my room or prohibited from watching TV.

Sometimes I felt that my parents favored her, but I am sure she thought that they favored me. In any event, they would deny it either way. They would also admonish us for feeling that way. To my parents, it was important that we felt as if we were being treated equally, but we seldom did. Whenever there was a disagreement, one or the other of us would complain that the solution "just wasn't fair."

Yet even as my sister and I grew into our teens and went our separate ways, there was an inexplicable bond between us. We didn't have to agree on things to be able to recognize what we meant to each other. We both acknowledged, even if at times reluctantly, that we were an important part of each other's lives.

As I grew older and adolescence led to generational disagreements, I still remained close to my parents. Navigating the minefield of adolescence often led to seeing the world differently. Whether we disagreed over my attempts to grow my curly brown hair longer or their obvious lack of enthusiasm for my musical selections, I always measured myself by the values I learned from

23

my family. Even heated discussions over the war in Vietnam never infringed on the true nature of our relationships. My strong family bonds created a basis for how I related to the rest of the world.

Energized with youth and optimism, I was ready to find out who I was and my place in the world. Eager to match my enthusiasm with deeds, I tamed my anxiousness of leaving home and tried to anticipate what life would be like away from family and friends. I didn't know what was in store for me but I was ready to find out. I am sure, to my mom and dad, I had grown up all too fast.

My parents left my education pretty much up to the "professionals," but the advice from the counselors at high school was practically non-existent. So when it came time to decide where to go to college, my choices were limited. I had a relative who sat down with me one Saturday to help me pick some schools. He asked my grades, looked in a book, and chose a college in Florida. I applied and was accepted.

Looking back, I suppose it was as random as monkeys throwing darts at stock picks. They win some and they lose some. Realistically, though, it was no way to determine what direction your life should go in.

Idealistic and filled with great expectations about the future, I left for college in early September. On the plane ride to Florida, I read a letter that my mom handed me right before I got on board:

September 1, 1970

Dear Larry,

    It's Saturday morning and tomorrow you'll be flying to Florida on your way to a new experience. It is a change we'll all have to adjust to. You take with you the strength, perseverance, and wisdom of your father; the affection and sentimentality of your mother; and all the love in the world from both of us. We are proud of the young man you have become. Now you face the future, and we know that you are truly equipped to accept the challenge.

Remember, we are as far away as a telephone call or letter. We are always here if you need us.

Love,
Mom and Dad

As I flew to Florida, I felt as if I carried the hopes and dreams my parents had for me.

Florida was a long way from home and I was pretty homesick at first. It wasn't as if it was my first experience away from home. One year, when we were younger, my parents sent Debbie and me off to sleep-away camp. Come to think of it, it was the same relative who helped me pick a college who thought camp would be a good idea too. Debbie and I were homesick and we ran away.

As I recall, it was actually Debbie who hatched the plan. I thought we could stick it out until visiting day. I was sure that we could convince my parents camp was a nice experiment that had gone awry and now it was time to come home. Debbie disagreed and was very determined to let me know how unhappy she was. I told her maybe if we call home, mom and dad will come pick us up. She reminded me that no one was allowed to make any telephone calls.

My mom told me that when Debbie was a baby and cried, I'd stick my thumb in her mouth to calm her down. So with Debbie overwrought and pining for home, her mind was set on leaving. I guess running away was my method of pacifying her. Besides, I was somewhat homesick too.

Our plan was to sneak out of camp right underneath the nose of the camp director whose headquarters guarded the front gate of the camp. We'd head down the turnpike to New York City, meet my father at his store, and our camp experience would be a short-lived memory. Excited about our plan, we both agreed it felt like we were about to embark on a great adventure. We wasted no time in activating our scheme. We gathered a few necessities, some cookies and Ring Dings, and off we went. When we made it past the front "command post," we felt as if we had pulled off the perfect caper.

We traveled as far as three miles, hiding behind a tree with every vehicle that passed. Then Debbie asked me, "Do you think there are any bears around?" Astonished at the reality of the question and considering the answer, I silently concluded maybe it wouldn't be such a bad idea if we got caught. I told Debbie that it was ridiculous to keep dodging cars. It would take us forever to get home. We brazenly ignored the next vehicle and happily it was the camp director and his assistant.

The camp director was pretty angry. After he drove us back to camp, he called our parents. I thought that maybe we'd get to go home after all. Unfortunately, he convinced my mom and dad that it would be best for us to remain in camp. We stayed the entire summer. I ended up liking it. I played a lot of baseball, swam in a lake, and kissed my first girl. Debbie, however, was contentious to the end.

My camp experience served me well when I found myself homesick again in my first month of college. I knew, in time, I would adjust. For now, though, I missed my friends and family back in New York.

I kept in touch with everyone mostly through the mail. There weren't telephones in the dorm room and calling home wasn't encouraged. Today college kids have phones, televisions, computers connected to the Internet, and every possible electronic device in their rooms. It seems pretty hard to imagine now, but at that time, calling home regularly was a luxury that my family couldn't afford. Besides an occasional call, we wrote to each other several times a week.

Visiting the campus post office became a daily ritual. It was a place filled with electricity and excitement. In between classes, everyone would file into the office to get the latest news from home or from a friend on another campus. Located next to an open courtyard, we would linger on the grass, opening letters and carefully examining postcards. New friends would exchange stories about the people back home and new bonds were formed. There were always a lot of smiles but occasionally someone would leave crying. In an instant, a buzz would go through the crowd usually giving sketchy details about a failed romance.

In my third week at school, I received a letter from my mom that began to detail what was to become the medical drama that would plague my sister for the rest of her life:

September 22, 1970

Dear Larry,

It's a warm and rainy Saturday morning and my thoughts are of you and how you are coming along. From the tone of your last letter, you seem to be managing nicely. Your father went to work and probably won't be home until late. He has been very busy lately and has no one to help him because your grandfather went on a vacation to the mountains.

Debbie has been ill since Wednesday. Dr. Gittleson

feels that she has a urinary tract infection, and he is treating her with antibiotics. Hopefully, it will clear up quickly. She has already started school, and I don't want her to miss too much work.

By the way, neither your father nor your sister wants your old job of throwing out the garbage. Put your mind at ease, your old job is securely waiting for you!

I look forward to your next letter.

Love,
Mom

A pretty routine letter, I thought. It sounded as if life was flowing normally back home, except for the fact that my mom couldn't find a recruit to dispose of the trash.

In the next couple of weeks, I received several letters from home–mostly from my mom and sister–but some from my father, too. There were increasing references to my sister not being well.

In part of one of her letters, Debbie wrote:

"Yesterday was some day! The TV went out, the car got towed, and the heat went out in the house. Mommy and Daddy were real frustrated.

Dr. Gittleson says I have a kidney infection called nephritis. I have to stay home from school for a few weeks and rest in bed. After that, I'll be okay. My body is swelling up. At first, I thought I was gaining weight but Dr. Gittleson says it's because of what's going on with my kidneys. I don't feel too bad but I'm more tired than usual."

My first reaction was that my sister must have found a new way of getting out of school. From a very early age, she was very clever at getting out of doing things she really didn't like. She would follow through on ideas that I could only dream of doing. Debbie was inventive in a lot of ways. Mostly, though, she had a rebellious spirit. Sometimes it enabled her to get what she wanted, but at other times, it got her into trouble.

I recall one particular New Year's Eve very vividly. My parents had gone out to celebrate the festivities with the Kleins, our next door neighbors. They left me in charge of Debbie and the Klein kids, Randy and Glenn. I was sixteen and Debbie was thirteen. Randy was a year younger than I was and Glenn was Debbie's age.

We all sat around the kitchen table gobbling up cocktail franks and soda. We were laughing and teasing each other. I hadn't noticed that Debbie was gone until she came into the room and went over to the utility cabinet. She quietly pulled out a hammer and tiptoed out of the kitchen. A split second later, I heard the front door creak open. I looked at Randy and Glenn. We all had a bewildered look on our faces. I sprung up and bolted out the door. Randy and Glenn were right behind me.

There, outside, was my sister banging the hammer against the side of my father's old big-finned Chrysler. "What the hell is going on?" I said aloud. Debbie stopped briefly to say she had an accident. "You what?" I shrieked. Before I could get an answer, she was whacking away at the car's fender again. "Debbie, stop for a second and tell me what happened."

"I took the car out for a ride and crashed it into a telephone pole."

"You took the car out for a ride?"

"Yeah, I know how to drive."

"Doesn't look that way to me."

"Very funny. Mommy and Daddy are going to kill me.

You've got to help me!" The Kleins stood there with goofy smiles, amazed at Debbie's deed. I grabbed the hammer away from Debbie and told them all to go back into the house.

I took one look at the crushed front end and knew we were in real big trouble. With hammer in hand, I launched a few swings at the aquamarine fender to no avail and went back into the house. What seemed like only moments later, my parents came walking up the steps. We could hear my father jingling his keys, an ominous sign that he was anxious to get through the front door. Debbie quickly retreated into her room. My father came in, and I saw immediately on his face that he had seen the wreckage. Unfortunately, Debbie had parked the car right under the street light.

"What did you do to the car?" he demanded. Since I had a learner's permit and was already taking Drivers Ed, I was the logical culprit. I hesitated–I couldn't get myself to tell him it was Debbie. As it turned out, I didn't have to. Debbie emerged from her room with a look of guilt and defiance in her eyes.

"Did you take the car out for a joy ride?" my father asked, half-amazed that he could consider the possibility.

"Yes," she said proudly, her chin jutting out defiantly halfway across the room.

"I don't believe you. You're covering up for your brother."

Well, eventually my parents believed that it was Debbie. Early the next morning, my father went out to see if there was a store open where he could buy a paper. He got as far as the front walk when he noticed that our other car had a flat tire on the left side.

It seems as if Debbie had taken both cars out that night. When the first car got a flat going around the block, she brought it home and immediately set sail in the second.

We both got in trouble that New Year's Eve, Debbie for her

escapades and me for not being a more diligent babysitter. Yet years later, that New Year's Eve story was often retold as family folklore. Invoking my sister's fabled ride was also a way of describing her mischievous make-up.

3

❖ ❖ ❖ ❖

As September ended and October began, the tone of the letters from home grew more concerned. My mother wrote that Debbie wasn't able to shake her infection, couldn't go back to school, and had to be tutored at home:

October 5, 1970

Dear Larry,

    Your letter came today and it's always a good feeling when we see a letter from you in the mailbox.

    Debbie is in the dining room making all kinds of grimaces at me. She is taking a French lesson and is obviously not too happy about it. Usually I leave the house, but I'm stuck here because my car wouldn't start this morning. So instead of suffering your sister's displeasure, I decided to write a quick note to you. If you get a chance, write to your grandma and grandpa. They are anxious to hear from you.

Love,
Mom

My father wrote that Debbie was giving them all a scare:

"She has some kind of kidney disorder but Gittleson doesn't think it's too bad. She'll have to go for additional testing though. Gittleson is determined to zero in on what's making her sick. She seems tired all the time."

I guess Debbie was sick after all. I still felt that everything would be okay because Dr. Gittleson always fixed up all the kids, whatever the problem. Whether it was chicken pox, measles, colds, or allergies, Dr. Gittleson always knew what to do. Whether it was medicine, a shot, or just staying home from school and resting in bed, he always took care of us and we always bounced back.

On October 12, 1970, my mom wrote:

Dear Larry,

It's Thursday. The weather is starting to change and the leaves are bright orange, yellow, and brown. It really looks beautiful on the trees. This year, your father will have to rake the leaves without you.

Debbie is still sick. At first, the doctor said he felt it was a urinary tract infection, then a kidney infection, but the medicine just wasn't completely helping her. So, yesterday we spent half the day at Dr. Gittleson's office taking more tests. He promises we'll know more in a few days when he calls with the results. Hopefully we'll get to the bottom of all this and Debbie will recover swiftly.

Please write soon. We all look forward to receiving your letters.

Love,
Mom

Meanwhile, life was changing for my sister.

On November 1, 1970, she wrote:

Dear Larry,

Hi, how are you? Well, I'm still a little sick. I've been out of school for six weeks. I thought I'd be back by now. As it looks, I probably won't be going back for at least another two weeks. I'm a little scared. It's going to be hard for me to get used to being in school again. All the kids are used to their teachers and each other. I'll feel like an outsider. I hope that my friends will help me out.

Anyway, I look forward to seeing you at Thanksgiving.

I love you and miss you,
Debbie

I tried to imagine what it was like for Debbie and my parents back home. I knew that my sister wasn't an easy patient when she was sick. Right about now, Debbie was probably insisting on playing a few rounds of Chinese checkers. In the early afternoon, my mom would most likely be running all over town trying to track down that one special treat that would put a smile on my sister's face. Then later, on his way home from work, I'm sure my father stopped at a restaurant to take out whatever culinary delight Debbie's palate yearned for that day.

After awhile, I started to get used to living in the dorms and steadily I became acclimated to college life on campus. Even though I found myself to be a champion procrastinator when it came time to doing laundry, I was adjusting to my newfound independence and responsibilities. I began to make friends and was even enjoying some of my classes. I still missed my family and friends back home, though, and kept corresponding with them by the mail. I looked forward to seeing everyone during the holiday.

Before I knew it, I was boarding a plane jam-packed with college students bound for Thanksgiving in New York. I thought that coming home for the holiday was wonderful. It was great to see my family and friends again. We were all excited to be with each other. There was lots of eating, of course, and even more hugs and kisses. Coming from sunny Florida, it was nice to see the change of season, too.

On Thanksgiving morning, I sat drinking hot chocolate and watching the leaves swirl in eddies in the backyard. My mom started cooking the night before and the house was filled with an aroma that said welcome home.

That afternoon, Debbie, my father, and I sat around the living room watching the early football game. We were patiently waiting for my grandparents, my aunt, uncle, and cousins to arrive. The three of us took turns running into the kitchen to see what we could nab from the kitchen table, which was beginning to fill up with the most delicious holiday treats.

It reminded me of when Debbie and I were little and my parents would have company. My mom would always fill bowls with assorted candies and nuts and pretzels and potato chips and popcorn, a virtual cornucopia of treats, all of which we weren't supposed to touch. But Debbie and I would stage raiding parties, grabbing whatever we could manage and then rearrange my mother's assortments. Several times in our zealousness to satisfy that can't-eat-just-one feeling, we miscalculated our take, leaving the bowls half empty.

This time my father joined us, doing his part quite nicely rearranging the carrots, celery, and cherry tomatoes, which were neatly posed around three exotic tangy dips.

Everyone arrived bringing different things. My aunt and uncle came in with an assortment of pies–pecan, pumpkin, and apple. One cousin brought her latest sweet potato concoction. My grandmother brought boxes of chocolates, cashew nuts, and assorted candies. My grandfather, as usual, brought his smelly cigar.

My grandmother immediately came in and before she even took off her coat, complained that my grandfather's cigar was stinking up the place. Debbie readily agreed. That was his signal to grab the dog's leash, turn right around, and take a quick stroll around the block to finish his cigar in peace. All the women headed for the kitchen and with an efficiency that would make a marine sergeant envious, the holiday meal was on its way to the dining room table. One dish after the other took its place until the table was filled with every available space occupied.

No one had to be asked twice to sit down. My grandfather must have sensed that dinner was being served because he was walking in the front door as my father was carving the turkey that had been roasting for half a day. I don't know who ran to the table faster, my grandfather or the dog.

Around the dinner table, the conversation revolved around school, business, and politics. That led to an emotional discussion over the war in Vietnam. My cousin and I had registered with the draft board early in the fall and it added a sense of realism to the conversation. With the tension level rising around the holiday table, my aunt changed the subject by asking Debbie how she was feeling. Everyone's attention shifted to Debbie and with some hesitation she said, " I'm doing all right. I should be going back to school soon."

That was all she said and the conversation swiftly changed again. Soon, there was a chorus of how everything was so delicious, how quickly we all ate, and how distressfully full we were.

After dinner, my grandma, mom, and aunt went into the kitchen to clean up. My grandfather headed for the door, cigar in one hand and the dog's leash in the other. Debbie and I, along with several of our cousins, went into the living room to talk and listen to music. My cousin, David, lobbied for Jefferson Airplane or Janice Joplin. His sister, Lynn, preferred Joni Mitchell and Judy Collins, while Debbie put on the full court press for anything Motown. She loved the beat of the Four Tops or the Temptations. I made convincing arguments for a compromise of either the Beatles or Crosby Stills Nash & Young.

My father and uncle were still sitting around the dinner table. While munching on cashews and arguing about the economy, they yelled to us to keep the music down. My uncle shook his head and said something like how can they listen to that music.

Before long, it was time for everyone to go home. With smiles and tears, we all said goodbye. We watched out the front window as everyone got into their cars and drove away.

With everyone gone, my mom went back into the kitchen to finish cleaning up, and my dad silently ran off to see if he could catch the end of the late afternoon football game. Debbie and I sat around the dining room table reminiscing about the day's events.

We laughed at how my grandfather had loosened his belt because he stuffed himself and then his pants began to fall down when he got up to leave the table. My grandmother was not amused and yelled at him, "Alfred, buckle up your pants." Everyone laughed hysterically, including my grandfather. Even my grandmother was coaxed into smiling. She tried unsuccessfully to hold herself back but immediately gave way to an infectious and generous giggle, which set everyone roaring.

Then, abruptly, Debbie said she wanted to go lie down because she was feeling tired. I asked, "Are you feeling all right?"

"I'm just tired. I'm not used to having so many people around."

"What's happening with you? Are you feeling any better?"

"I don't know what to think. Sometimes I feel better, but at other times, I don't feel right at all."

Debbie got up and slowly walked across the living room and down the hall, vanishing into her room. After she left, I went into the kitchen and asked my mom what was happening with Debbie's infection. Without looking up from drying the dishes, she said that she was concerned because Dr. Gittleson still wasn't sure what was wrong. The testing showed that she had an infection, but Dr. Gittleson didn't know what was causing it. There were still some additional tests he wanted to run. She didn't say much after that except to say with a sigh, "I'm hoping that before too long, your sister will be all right." Then she shifted gears by asking me if I had met any girls at school. I told her I had met several nice girls I considered friends but not anyone I thought of as a "girlfriend."

The Thanksgiving holiday was over too soon, and like thousands of other college kids, I boarded a plane and headed back to life in the dorms. It was really great to see everybody again. I knew I was coming home for Christmas vacation and looked forward to spending more time in New York. While Debbie seemed more tired than usual, my four day trip back home didn't give me any clue of what was to follow.

It wasn't long after I arrived back at school that I received a surprising letter from my mother:

December 2, 1970

Dear Larry,

Good morning! We have another rainy day and it's unseasonably warm. It's 8:35 in the morning and Debbie is still sleeping. Dr. Gittleson just called. He wants her to go into the hospital for more tests. He said it could be a couple of days or even a week before a bed becomes available. He's making all the arrangements. I just wish all the tests were over and Debbie was done with all this.

Love,
Mom

I was pretty surprised to hear that Debbie had to go into the hospital for the testing. Suddenly the uncertainty of her situation heightened my awareness that this was more than a typical infection. The same day, I also received a letter from Debbie that she had written later that day.

Dear Larry,

> Dr. Gittleson is putting me in the hospital for these tests and I'm getting very scared. He's put me on a strict diet–all I can eat is cottage cheese and peaches and things like that. Larry, I'm so bored at home. The last few days I've had to stay in bed all the time. I'm gaining weight, and I'm tired and moody. I've been weak lately and now Mommy and Daddy don't want me to go out at all.
>
> I've been scheduled for a biopsy next week. I never heard of a biopsy before but it's where they take a small tissue sample of the kidney. They get it by putting a needle into the kidney and pulling out a piece of tissue through the needle. Then they're going to study the sample and see what's going on in my kidneys. The whole thing gives me the creeps. Write back soon.
>
> Love,
> Debbie

It gave me the creeps, too. I remember putting down Debbie's letter and thinking that poor Debbie probably doesn't know what to think. Several days later, I received another letter from my mom:

December 5, 1970

Dear Larry,

It's Saturday morning and I'm getting ready to visit Debbie in the hospital. They're constantly taking blood and urine and measuring her blood pressure. Debbie says she's starting to feel like a pincushion. On Monday or Tuesday, they'll be doing a biopsy. The day they admitted her was a day filled with tension and apprehension. Debbie was really very brave and mature and made things easier on me and made me proud of her. I hope all is well with you.

Love
Mom

From Debbie's letter, it was easy to see that she was afraid. Who wouldn't be? My mom wrote about how proud she was of her and so was I. I felt very distant from the situation, though. There was nothing I could do to help. All I could do was wait.

4

❖ ❖ ❖ ❖

"Larry, Molly, come on up for breakfast." Carolyn called to us out the kitchen window, which overlooks the backyard. " Josh is up and I'm making pancakes for us."

"I guess she's finished taking a shower, girl," I said to Molly. Her head tilted to one side as I spoke.

"I'm not hungry."

"Larry, I think you should eat something. Yesterday I went out and bought that special pure maple syrup you like."

"Maybe I'll come up in a little while."

"At least let me bring you a glass of juice or something."

"Maybe later."

"Josh is getting dressed. He wants to know if you videotaped Star Trek for him last night."

"I put it in his room on his desk."

"That will make him happy," she said. "Now make me happy and come in and join us for breakfast."

"I'm fine. You two enjoy the pancakes and I'll eat something later."

"All right, let Molly in and at least I'll feed her," Carolyn said.

Upon hearing her name, Molly was already waiting at the door to be let in. She looked back at me wagging her tail as if to say, "Let's get going before it's all gone." So without making her wait a moment longer, I got up and let her in. She bolted in the house and up the stairs. She momentarily stopped at the landing, looking back at me to see if I was coming. I waved her on and said, "Go ahead, breakfast is waiting."

"What a wonderful life I have," I said to myself, thinking about Molly running upstairs to join Carolyn and Josh. Who could want anything more? Carolyn and I have been married for eighteen fulfilling years. Our son, Josh, who just turned thirteen, is our heart's delight.

I stood there for a moment and looked around the yard. With my heart filled with gratitude and tender thoughts of my family, I went back to my chair, sat down, and allowed the sun to wash over me once again. Within seconds, the light seemed to fill every cell of my being. I closed my eyes, breathed deeply, and accepted the sun's warmth. I could hear the soft aria of a lone cardinal in the willow tree. Now, almost in a meditative trance, my mind shifted beyond my surroundings; and I found myself again recounting the narrative about my sister.

I decided to call Debbie's hospital room on Tuesday to find out what was happening. After a few rings, my mom answered the phone. Speaking softly into the receiver, she whispered that they had done the biopsy and Debbie was finally resting comfortably. Now we had to wait for the results.

Two days later, right after my late morning biology class and before lunch, I made my daily pilgrimage to the campus post office. I was expecting some news about Debbie. The PO, as it was called, was unusually calm for that time of day. I went directly to my mail slot, looked into the little window and saw a blue envelope with white masking tape sealing the edges. I immediately recognized Debbie's stationery and her tamperproof fastening method. I stumbled through the combination, opened the box, and retrieved her letter.

As I stood in front of the wall of mailboxes, I read about Debbie's experience. As usual, reading her handwriting was like trying to decipher an encrypted code.

December 10, 1970

Dear Larry,

I am writing to you from the hospital. Mommy and Daddy told me that you called when I was sleeping. I was in a lot of pain from the biopsy. Even though the doctor sedated me a little, I was still fully aware of what was happening. They had an X-ray machine monitoring dye that was going through my bloodstream and into the kidneys. Once it reached the kidneys, the doctor saw where to position the needle to take out the tissue sample. Suddenly, I felt a jabbing in my back. It was the pressure from where he put in the needle into the kidney. When it was over, I returned to my room and had to lay flat on my back for a day. When I finally got out of bed, I was in a lot of pain. They say we will have the results in about a week.

Larry, I'm afraid. I don't know what's happening to me. I wish you were here. I miss you.

Love,
Debbie

I was pretty stunned to hear the details of what Debbie had to go through. I never knew anyone so sick that he or she needed anything like a biopsy. I remember kids with broken arms and all of us had the usual assortment of childhood diseases and viruses—but not anything like this.

I slowly walked out of the post office rereading Debbie's letter to make sure I didn't misread anything. With each step, I tried to gain a sense of what was happening to my sister, but I really didn't know what to think.

The following week, I decided to call my parents to see if they heard the results of the biopsy. They weren't home, but my sister picked up the phone.

"Debbie, how are you doing? Did you here from the doctors yet?" I asked.

"We just heard about an hour ago."

"What did they say?"

"They analyzed the tissue and said that there has been damage to both my kidneys. They felt medicine would stop the damage from continuing, and I could live on the remaining undamaged portion of my kidneys."

"Where are Mom and Dad?" I asked.

"They went over to the doctor's office to get the prescription for the medicine. The doctors want me to get started on it right away to prevent any further damage."

"How are you, Debbie?

"I'm still not feeling very well. I'm always tired and achy."

"Were you scared when they did the biopsy?" I asked.

"I was a little nervous."

"How do you feel now?"

"When I first came home, I kind of missed the hospital. Crazy as it might seem, I missed the security of the people caring for me."

"Well, they're good places to stay out of, Deb."

"Now you sound like Mommy,"

"Well, Mom's right."

"I'm only telling you how I feel."

"That's okay. I'm just glad that the doctors figured out what's wrong with you, and they can give you medicine that will help."

"I hope so. They want to see me and do testing once a month to monitor how I'm doing. I wish this whole thing was over."

"Me too, Deb."

"Well, I have to go. Tell Mommy and Daddy I called. I'll write to you soon."

"Okay, Larry, thanks for calling. I'll keep writing to you. We all miss you, including the dog."

"I miss all of you, too."

With that, we hung up.

In a way, I felt relieved. It seemed as if the doctors found out what was wrong with Debbie and they had a way of controlling it. But she still wasn't feeling good and no one could tell us if that was going to change.

5

❖ ❖ ❖ ❖

My first year in college was over before I knew it. While I was away, the frequent letters and occasional calls kept me informed about how Debbie was doing, but they didn't prepare me for what that actually meant. When I came home for summer vacation, the world had changed dramatically. Life as I knew it was gone. Though my parents were happy that I was home, they were noticeably subdued. Debbie's spirits were vanquished. Being ill for the entire year was wearing very thin. I had left a vibrant family and returned to an air of discouragement.

My parents decided to put an in-ground swimming pool in the backyard, hoping to raise Debbie's spirits. My sister had spent the entire fall and winter isolated at home. My mom and dad felt that a pool would allow her to have friends over and not be so alone. They also thought that it would be a wonderful way for all of us to enjoy being together during the summer.

I can't say that I was very happy with the idea at first. I was concerned that I would miss the trees I climbed as a boy, especially the one my cousin David tried to chop down with a croquet mallet while practicing his role in the fourth grade school play as Paul Bunyan.

Soon, however, music and poolside barbecues, along with a constant parade of friends and relatives, made it a summer to remember. The scent of suntan lotion filled the air, and if you closed your eyes, you'd think you were at the beach. While sipping lemonade and iced tea, a soft night breeze soothed the day's heat. When it was time to go to sleep, you could hear the pool jets playing a soothing melody from the open window that gently lulled us to sleep.

While Debbie's disease was never far from view, that summer by the pool was an oasis. Unfortunately, it was also a mirage. With the onset of fall and the new school year, Debbie found herself sequestered again. Her friends went back to school and she began the year with home tutors.

During the summer, I decided to leave school in Florida and continue with my education in New York. In September, I transferred to Pace University in New York City. I wanted to be closer to my family. I commuted into the city and lived at home. Traveling on the Long Island Railroad was a far cry from being in Florida and walking across campus to class in balmy 70-degree weather. It still amazes me how easy it was to fall into the commuter's lament. The dash to catch an early morning train also meant invoking the power of prayer in the hunt for a parking space. After a brief pause celebrating the good fortune of finding a space for your car, the next order of business was finding a seat on a packed commuter train. The grand prize was to find a place where you could park yourself in an effort to read or take a snooze.

Even though I complained as any good commuter would, most of the time it felt as if I was really playing at riding the rails. I was primarily fascinated by the diversity of so many different kinds of people, all making their way to New York City. I wondered about who they were. What was their life like? How different they all looked, all seeming to play a unique part in the drama of life.

While I spent time studying the history of the Ming dynasty of China at the university, and imagined the lives of my fellow road warriors, my sister's difficulties continued. My mother ferried back and forth to the hospital with Debbie for constant tests that measured her kidney function. With every visit, I would ask how she was doing. The answer was always that nothing had changed–maybe she was a little better.

I knew, though, that things were not really improving. My sister spent a lot of time sleeping in a silent, dark room all day. She became very sensitive to noise and light. The curtains were always closed. I would have to tiptoe around the house for fear of disturbing her resting in the dark living room. In the corner, a baby grand piano stood silent. Once it filled the air with the most delightful sounds of my mother playing Mozart and Chopin. Even the not-so-melodic tune of two children practicing their scales was sadly gone. Our house was becoming morbid.

Times also change. Families grow and houses become too small. Careers are recast and families and friends drift apart. My mom's sister moved her family to Connecticut and my parents' best friends and next door neighbors moved to New Jersey. It seemingly served as a reminder that life was going on for other people, while my parents found themselves trapped and derailed from their intended course.

Other friends and relatives didn't know what to say and some stopped calling altogether. Debbie's disease was beginning to take its toll on all of us. My parents hardly went out anymore and were beginning to find themselves isolated. We were all becoming

51

hostages to Debbie's illness.

It was as if we were all waiting for something to happen. Somehow I felt that things were going to turn around. I thought that ultimately, Debbie was going to be all right. Maybe it was the optimism of youth, or maybe I just didn't want to face the alternative of Debbie being like this for the rest of her life. I thought that either the medication would kick in or maybe someone would discover a new medication to help her.

While I hoped for change, life was becoming fractured. Living at home was not as I imagined it would be when I transferred back to New York. Often, I would come home from school and Debbie would be trying to sleep in the living room because she was feeling fatigued or because she had a headache. Almost daily, my mom would meet me at the entranceway and usher me into my room so Debbie could rest. Most of the time I understood, but I became increasingly frustrated to be banished to a small corner of our home.

The vitality around the kitchen table at dinnertime was replaced with quiet, sullen meals. After dinner, we would all go our separate ways. I would retreat to my room, close the door, and quietly do homework. If I made plans with a friend, we'd have to meet somewhere because people coming to the house would often disturb the delicate balance of unobtrusive silence that Debbie required. I began to feel disconnected.

In May, I decided to transfer to a school away from home. I don't really remember all the details or reasons, but I am sure that part of the reason was that I wanted to get away from the air of desolation that pervaded my home.

Sometimes, I think that I had to get away because I felt guilty that I was healthy and Debbie wasn't. Happiness seemed to be a feeling that was exiled from our lives. Any of life's celebrations were placed in suspended animation. The expression of personal joy became a stigma infused with shame and guilt.

I knew that Debbie was sick, but I thought that she was eventually going to be okay. So I didn't always understand why everything seemed to be so grave. I didn't understand until recently, when I learned that my parents knew very early on that Debbie wasn't going to get better. They knew from the results of the biopsy. The doctors informed them that Debbie had a degenerative disease that slowly and steadily would cause complete kidney failure. The medicine she took was an attempt to forestall the inevitable. Debbie's life was in jeopardy all along. My parents decided that it was best not to tell us.

Looking back, I'm sure they wanted Debbie and me to live a normal life. On one hand, I wished they had confided in me about the severity of the situation. If I knew, maybe it would have made a difference in understanding what my parents and Debbie were going through. If I knew that things were so serious, maybe I would have better understood some of the emotions that were flying around. Maybe I wasn't supportive enough. Perhaps I would have stayed home to help out. I questioned whether I should have been protected like that.

On the other hand, I understand their decision not to tell us. Ultimately, they tried to give me a gift. They wanted me to experience college and all the joys of that magical time unbound by the full worry I would have felt if I had known. It's funny how two sides of an issue can be so different, yet both can be valid.

I realized that keeping a secret like that from their children could not have been an easy thing for my parents. Very few people knew how truly critical Debbie's situation was. My parents only revealed how desperate their circumstances were to a few close friends and relatives. Most people knew that Debbie was very sick, but they didn't know that her life was threatened. Now, I wonder how many suspected.

Even though the doctors told my parents in no uncertain terms that Debbie was in mortal danger, my mom and dad still held out hope that her life could be prolonged enough that perhaps a new medication, a change in diet, or something would reverse the decree. My father would call home several times a day from work to see if there was any change. "Is she feeling any better? Is she as lethargic as yesterday?" Everyday my mom would give him the disappointing news. "No real change, maybe things will be better this afternoon." The next day would come and it would be the same refrain. And so their days would go for the next three years.

6

❖ ❖ ❖ ❖

I transferred from Pace University in New York City to the State University of New York at New Paltz. I left home again in the fall with several friends that had also transferred. I was excited to embark on a new adventure. Debbie was just about to begin her senior year in high school. Considering that she was home tutored and out of school so often, it was surprising that she didn't lose any ground in school.

It was a good year for me. I lived in the dorms, met a lot of nice people, did well in school, and generally felt alive. New Paltz was a rural village surrounded by small but captivating mountains whose beauty celebrated the hue of every season.

Hiking the highlands in the fall revealed the most dazzling array of color that I had ever seen. I wasn't just an audience to the various shades of red–cherry, rose, and ruby. In some discernable way, I was participating with every tint of brown, every cast of yellow, and every orange tinge. Every tone of green–forest, lime, olive, jade, and emerald–vibrated through me completely over-whelming my senses.

I was hypnotized by the silent splendor of walking down a country road at sunrise. As the wind would whisper through the tall grass, the rhythm of my own breath quickly joined the seething sounds of the early morning. The rise and fall of the cricket's call harmonized with the crackling of leaves stirred by the onset of a westerly breeze. All things merged in song, as if announcing the arrival of a new day.

At nighttime, the sky shimmered. There were so many stars that lit the evening, it was impossible not to feel the wonder of it all. In some way, the stars reminded me of last year and how all the different people riding the railroad were unique, yet a part of some grander portrait. I couldn't help but marvel at how each star also seemed distinct, yet all of them together weaved a gleaming mosaic, an infinite tapestry streaking across the evening sky.

I delighted in my new surroundings, but my concern for my sister and parents was never far below the surface. I would always call home to find out how things were. When I asked about Debbie, the answer was always the same: she's doing okay. Debbie's illness had become a given. It was an ever-present fact of life that didn't seem to have a resolution.

This changed in the spring of that year. After three years, my parents finally told me the full scope of my sister's illness.

It was early April and I was home for the weekend. An unusually warm Sunday morning made it ideal for lounging around in the backyard. Trying to rush the coming of summer, I poured a cool glass of lightly sweetened iced tea, grabbed the portable radio, and ensconced myself outside in a most agreeable deck chair. I had just turned on the radio and started to flip through the stations when my father called to me, "Larry, come into the house for a moment. Your mom and I would like to talk to you about something." Oh damn, I thought! I knew I shouldn't have had my friends over last night. My father must have found the bottle of Chablis in the garbage. Oh well, it wasn't the first time.

"What's up?" I asked, walking through the dining room. "Please sit down. We have something to talk to you about." "What's the matter?" "It's about your sister." "Where is Debbie anyway? I didn't see her this morning."

I think my question was an attempt to delay some dreadful news that I intuitively felt was about to be unleashed. "She went over to Betty's house. The two of them are taking her baby sister to the swings in the park."

"Larry, Debbie's sick," my dad began. The next few moments, his words seemed to hang in the air, a dense thicket of information and emotion to wade through.

Debbie's kidneys were steadily and surely deteriorating. She had acute nephritis, which meant that in time, her kidneys would not function and she would lose the use of her kidneys completely.

My father explained that over the years, the doctors had tried several medications in an attempt to thwart the inevitable, all to no avail. There was no medical cure. When she lost kidney function altogether, she would die. The doctors could prolong her life by putting her on a dialysis machine. Dialysis meant being hooked up to a machine that mimics kidney function by purifying blood, but it is often painful and psychologically debilitating, especially for someone Debbie's age.

I looked at my mom, her eyes tearing, then at my Dad, whose concern washed over me like a heat wave rising off the summer's pavement.

All my parents' hopes for a miraculous turnaround were gone. They told me that Debbie's condition had worsened and she was already close to losing kidney function altogether. Soon, she would have to go on dialysis just to stay alive. The news was staggering. How could this happen? I asked my parents why the doctors couldn't do something.

My mom looked at my dad and he looked back to her. After what seemed like an unbearable pause, he continued.

There was something else that could be done to save Debbie's life. He said there was a possibility of Debbie getting a new kidney. It was a relatively new procedure that had yielded varying degrees of success. A donor kidney was required. The doctors said there were two sources for kidney donation. One source is from someone who just died and had previously agreed to allow his or her kidneys to be removed upon death for transplantation. This was called a cadaver donor. I have to admit, I thought it sounded a little gross.

Then my mom picked up the baton from my father and continued. The second option is a live donor transplant. She said someone, usually a family member, has one of his or her kidneys removed and transplanted into the person who needs it. I sat there, eyes widened and astonished at the possibility. I immediately wondered whether one of my parents would give Debbie a kidney.

My mom told me a successful transplant would be greatly enhanced coming from a brother, sister, or parent. Once I heard brother or sister, I began to realize that this situation could possibly include me. My mom concluded by saying that they were going to meet with Dr. Williams to get all the details, and I was welcome to come. My father touched his fingers to his forehead, holding his head as if it were a burden weighed down with too much to consider.

I sat there speechless, then whispered softly, " I can't believe all this," neither of my parents hearing. Then my mom asked me if I had any questions about the whole thing. I just sat there, simultaneously shrugging my shoulders and shaking my head no. We all looked at each other in a hushed silence.

With nothing left to say, I dragged myself off the couch and said that I wanted to go outside in the back and relax before the trip back to school. Half dazed, I spent the next few hours in the yard staring at a crystal blue sky, my mind unsuccessfully trying to grasp onto a single thought. Everything seemed blurred. Yesterday life seemed in place. Now it felt tossed and tangled.

During my April break from school, I went with Debbie and my parents to talk to Dr. Williams. He welcomed us into his small, well-kept office. After we walked in, he sat behind an imposing large oak desk with a protective glass top. On the corner was a stack of folders neatly arranged with different color labels. In back of him was a bookshelf tightly packed with periodicals and medical references. He invited us all to sit down. Debbie and I sat directly across from him in two oversized chairs, and my parents sat on a leather sofa on the right side of the room.

I felt a little awkward at first. My parents and Debbie already knew Dr. Williams and liked him very much. There was something about him that was calming and reassuring. Perhaps it was his grandfatherly white hair or maybe it was his easy manner. Yet at the same time, his steely blue eyes underscored a seriousness not to be taken lightly.

He asked Debbie how she was feeling. She told him she was tired and woozy. He said that she was going to have to get started on dialysis soon. Debbie didn't show her emotions readily; but when I looked over at her, I could tell she was scared. Dr. Williams said, "Don't worry; we'll get you through it."

Then he took a deep breath and immediately addressed all of us. "As you know, Debbie has acute nephritis. Over the last three years, her kidney function has steadily diminished." We all listened with resignation. "Now it's time we look at a relatively new surgery. It's where a new kidney is transplanted into someone whose kidneys are failing."

Dr. Williams went on to reiterate what my parents had already discussed with me. He told us that this was my sister's only hope.

Then Dr. Williams said something that surprised all of us, and I knew would change my life. He said, "Though our experience is somewhat limited, certain patterns are beginning to emerge. Nationally, so far it seems that a brother or a sister matches better than either parent." "What does that mean?" I said, startled, as my mind was seized by Dr. Williams' pronouncement.

"It means that if you and your family decide that a live donor is a possibility, then all of you will undergo extensive testing to decide whose kidney would give your sister the best chance of a successful transplant. However, there is a good chance that you'll be the best match."

I said I didn't understand. "Don't you just take out a kidney from one of us and hook it up in Debbie?"

"Basically that's what we do. However, the human body is a funny thing. The body of the person receiving the new kidney looks at it as a foreign object. It looks at the new kidney as something to repel. The body's defense mechanisms immediately spring into action and fight to rid itself of this perceived foreign invader. What it comes down to is that the body rejects the new kidney."

Then he continued. "Through trial and error, we have come to realize that to maximize our chance of success, we have to match the blood and tissue type, among other factors, of both the donor and the recipient. By doing that, we try to trick the recipient's body into thinking that the new kidney belongs there." He also added that even with a close match, Debbie would need to take drugs that would suppress her immune system so that her body would not reject the new kidney.

Then Dr. Williams directed his attention to me. Measuring his words, he repeated that even though there haven't been many transplants done nationally, experience indicates that a brother or sister matches better than either parent. "To date, a sibling seems to be our best hope for a successful transplant."

Suddenly I felt as if everyone in the room was looking at me and waiting for my reaction. The room was silent only for a brief moment, but I could feel the stillness seep through my skin.

I briefly glanced at my sister, who appeared unreadable. I then asked the doctor,

"You've been saying that your experience in kidney transplants is limited, right?"

"That's correct," he said.

"How many transplants have you done?" I asked.

"Well, we've done a number of transplants using cadaver donors. However, we've never had a live donor. We're hoping that your family will be the first."

All at once, it clicked, like a movie playing itself out. Past events seemed to line up like the pieces of a puzzle. Everything over the past few years magnetized to this defining moment.

I flashed back to the campus post office and all the letters detailing how Debbie first got sick. I remembered watching her lying on the couch in a silent, dark room, trying to hold back the disease that was speeding through her veins–seeing my home and the life of my family slowly, over the course of years, falling into an abyss of isolation and despair. Looking back at it now, I can't help but wonder: Was this destined to be?

I felt a rush of childhood memories. Debbie was my kid sister for who, from the beginning, I had both feelings of responsibility and competition. She wouldn't let me go out and play football with the guys unless I brought her with me. We made snow forts together and defended them against other neighborhood kids. In summertime, we'd giggle ourselves silly, as we cooled ourselves running through an icy-cold sprinkler in our bare feet. We fought and argued over who owned what record album. Once I even caught her trying to write her name on every record album as if that would establish her claim to our entire collection. We shared memories of holidays spent with cousins and grandparents. The two of us laughed and schemed. We argued about who would sit in the front seat of the car and who got to pick whether we would go bowling or to the movies.

Here was my sister who, in one instant, would take my side in an argument with my parents and then, in another, turn around and complain that I wouldn't let her into my room. Here she was, my younger sister, who, after years of distress, was now in such a desperate bind.

In an instant, I saw my future. Debbie needed a kidney transplant to save her life and I was going to be that donor. There was no doubt about it. This was my fate. I could feel it in my bones.

I felt everything at once. I could feel courage well up inside. Yet I wondered about the risks to me. Was I going to have to be put out? Was the surgery going to hurt? How long would it take to recover? Could I live with one kidney? Would it shorten my life? More and more questions came to mind.

My father broke the spell. He asked Dr. Williams to review the positives and negatives about cadaver donors versus a live donation from the family. I immediately thought that maybe I wouldn't have to do it after all. I had forgotten all about that possibility. This was quickly dispelled though, when the doctor said that at best, there was a sixty-percent chance of success with a cadaver kidney and a ninety-percent chance of success with a good match from a member of the family. To add to that difficulty, he further explained that there was a long list of people waiting for cadaver kidneys. He said that besides the wait, if a cadaver transplant was not successful, Debbie would have to wait for another kidney. She would then have to go through the surgery again. Dr. Williams finished by saying, "It's wise to go with your best chance first."

My mother and father immediately decided to take the necessary blood tests. They turned to me and told me that I didn't have to decide right away. They said that they didn't want me to feel that I had to do this.

Of course, I quickly agreed that taking the blood tests was the right thing to do. It was decided that we would all take the tests and wait to see the results. Then we would settle on what to do. Before we left Dr. Williams' office, he set up an appointment for us to do the necessary genetic testing. As I walked out of his office, I felt light-headed and unsure of the ground beneath my feet.

7

❖ ❖ ❖ ❖

"Larry, we're finished with breakfast. Are you coming up soon?" Carolyn called out the window, interrupting my voyage into the past.

"I'll be up in a little while."

"Are you sure you're okay? You sound so far away."

"I suppose I am. I was just thinking about the day I heard that Debbie was going to need a transplant. I just can't believe after all these years that this could happen now."

"I know, it's hard to accept, but life doesn't always go as we expect it to," she said.

Not saying anything, I shook my head in agreement.

"You want to take a ride with me to the store to get some groceries? We ran out of milk and I need a few other things besides."

"No, I'll wait in the backyard until you come back."

"You sure you don't want to come? It might take your mind off of it."

"No thanks."

"All right, then, I'm off. I'll tell Josh you're in the backyard just in case he needs you. He's in his room watching TV."

"Okay."

After having her fill of pancakes, Molly rejoined me and was sitting by my side carefully watching two squirrels chase after each other around the trunk of an old birch tree. Her interest heightened as one of the squirrels jumped to the ground. She leaped to her feet and was about to chase the little creature out of her territory, when it left of its own accord. "Good girl, Molly, you sure scared that squirrel away," I said. She jogged over to where it boldly crossed her territory. Then she sniffed around and decided to bark for good measure. With a job well done, she ran over to me, wagged her tail, and sat down by my side again. I gave her a pat on the head and said, "You're a good girl, Molly." Smiling at her antics, I quietly returned to my backyard musing.

My junior year in college was finally over. I came back home unsure of what the future would hold. It was a late June day. A warm breeze carried a decidedly floral fragrance, green and grassy. The maple trees and cherry blossoms swayed, swerving and bending ever so easily. The air was so agreeable you could practically taste its bouquet.

My father had gone to work later than usual and we all had breakfast together. Everyone seemed unusually animated. It was as if the optimism of spring filtered through the desperation of our situation. I don't exactly know why; maybe that's just what spring does to you.

My mom and sister excitedly made plans to go to the store to buy summer clothes. Amazingly, I almost had my father convinced to go fishing, but at the last minute he changed his mind. Not even the spontaneity of spring could break through my father's conscientious devotion to his business.

My dad went off to work and Debbie and my mom were off to the store. As an afterthought and I'm sure with little expectations of me saying yes, they invited me to come along. Anyway, I didn't have anything to do, so surprising even myself, I went for the ride.

It was a short, pleasant trip. We had the windows wide open and the air rushing in swept wildly through our hair. The radio rumbled with the latest hit songs, one right after the other. The music rolled on without interruption. We all felt emancipated, shaking our heads up and down and from side to side. Snapping our fingers to the beat, we were momentarily riding a boundless wave of freedom. The constant worry of Debbie's situation was temporarily lifted. It was a very welcome pause.

The excursion to the store was brief and we were back in about an hour and a half. The only thing that my mom and sister bought was a pair of brown sandals for each of them. I bought a magazine and a pack of gum from the newspaper stand.

When we returned, Debbie and my mom went into the house excited about their new purchases. I saw that the mailbox was full so I grabbed the mail and brought it in. Looking it over, there were the usual advertisements and bills. There was a letter from my aunt to my mom. Then I noticed the letter from the hospital.

We all knew it was coming, but I didn't expect it so soon. I guess I tried to push it out of my mind. My mother had confided in me that she thought for sure that she would be the match. She began to watch her health very closely and had become vigilant about what she ate. She was determined that her kidney be strong, thereby giving Debbie the greatest chance of a successful transplant.

I gave my mom the letter. She briefly inspected the envelope, looked at me, and then broke the seal. Deep down inside, I knew it was the official word that I matched my sister's blood and tissue type. I was going to be declared the winner in the sweepstakes to give my sister a kidney.

I have to admit that as my mother opened the letter, I secretly hoped that I wouldn't be the one. I also felt guilty for feeling that way. Sure enough, I wasn't only the best match, but I was "the perfect match." Neither my mom nor my dad came close to matching.

My parents spent the next couple of weeks assuring me that no one would think less of me if I chose not to go through with it. In my mind, though, there wasn't any choice. How could I live with myself if I didn't do this? My sister needed this to survive. I wasn't going to turn my back on her. Even though I was scared, I felt brave at the same time. I felt courageous, a gallant would-be hero, but I also felt like running away from what I knew I had to do.

All these contradictory emotions ran around in my head and heart. Ultimately, though, I loved my sister and my family. I was brought up to watch out for my younger sister. Was it because of the way I was brought up or was it part of my basic nature? I can't answer. All I know is that it was there and in an odd way, this was a logical expression of that impulse. The possibility of saying no was beyond any deductive reasoning, as well as emotional soul-searching.

The funny thing about it was that, even though I loved my sister, sometimes I felt close to her and at other times I didn't. Often, I felt that we were on different wavelengths. Judging by other families, our relationship was that of ordinary brother and sister. Sometimes we fought. Yet at other times, we got along, especially when we needed each other as allies against "parental tyranny." My relationship with my sister sure seemed ordinary.

At least it was until now.

Strangely, my sister and I barely spoke about the transplant. I would do it and she would accept it. There was very little discussion. I also remember that my sister wasn't exactly gushing over with appreciation. In fact, she made sure I knew that she wasn't going to treat me any differently. She said, "I'm still going to yell at you when you come into my room uninvited, and I'm ready and willing to argue and fight about who gets to play what record on the stereo."

Surprisingly, after our initial conversations, my parents also didn't talk to me much about the transplant. It's almost as though they felt that if we don't say anything, it will be done and over and we can get on with our lives. Perhaps they didn't know what to say. Life had handed them this situation without a road map–a daughter whose only chance for life was a transplant and a healthy son who was putting his life at risk. Both children were to be put in harm's way.

That summer, I spent most of the time swimming. In marked contrast to the last few summers, all our attempts to ascend beyond our dilemma fell short. I told some of my closest friends that I was going to give Debbie a kidney. Most of them said they would do it for their brother or sister. I remember thinking at the time how easy it was for them to say it when they didn't have to do it.

I also remember that most of my friends didn't really want to talk about it. They always seemed to be so uncomfortable whenever I would try to discuss it and that made me uncomfortable too. I began to feel that maybe it was me. Maybe it's just one of those things that everyone thinks is better kept to yourself. It seemed odd to me because I always thought that I could talk about anything with my friends. I quickly realized that I was left pretty much alone to sort out all the emotions I was feeling.

In spite of my family's muted reaction, I knew that I would have to get a handle on the situation. My mind flew, and I had many different thoughts. In some of my expansive moments, I imagined myself a hero in an adventure. I knew I was doing a courageous thing. How many people are asked to do this? At other times, I thought myself foolish and selfish for feeling that way. This was a matter of life and death and I'm fantasizing about being a hero. Besides, no one else seemed to be looking at me like one. I was mostly met with silence.

As the summer months passed, I became pensive. My fantasies lost their luster as the medical realities entered my thoughts. I was only twenty years old and had never had any surgery. What if the doctors made a mistake during surgery and something went wrong? I didn't want to end up physically disabled.

I remember several times thinking what if everything went wrong and I died? Every time I did, though, I quickly passed it off as some vague improbability. I suppose that at the age of twenty, you just don't see it happening to you, no matter what the circumstances. I guess I figured if I died, I died. I wouldn't know about it.

I also remember thinking of the possibility of giving Debbie a kidney and the transplant not working. This was one of the most distressing thoughts. I would have gone through all this for nothing, and what would Debbie do then? How pointless that would be, but then again, Debbie's sickness seemed pointless too.

I was determined to extinguish my doubts and look at everything in a positive vein. Nothing was going to go wrong. Debbie was going to get a new kidney. I was going to be fine. I would have the satisfaction of knowing that I was able to save my sister's life and that was all I really wanted. I was somewhat bewildered, though, about how quiet my parents and Debbie were about the whole thing. It was as if talking about it would break a code of silence or repeal some unspoken bargain.

The summer drew to a close and I made plans to go back to school. It was my last year, and in June, I would graduate. Graduation seemed like a decade away. Emotionally, the upcoming transplant infused everything I did and every thought I had, like an under-current that wouldn't let go.

Going back to school offered little comfort from my inner conversation. Walking down by a winding stream in the woods and watching the sunlight perform a flickering dance by the water's edge would sometimes soothe my mind.

Life kept moving on. Time didn't stop; it marched steadily on. It held the promise of uncertainty. It loomed as a borderline and a barrier to hurdle.

8

❖ ❖ ❖ ❖

Soon after I left for my senior year in school, Debbie began experiencing dizzy spells. My sister decided not to tell anybody how sick she was until one morning, she couldn't get out of bed. My parents rushed her to the hospital. The doctors took some blood tests, which revealed that Debbie's blood was being poisoned. Her kidneys had failed completely. She was going to have to go on dialysis and the transplant would have to be scheduled soon.

The doctors wanted me to be of legal age before they would go ahead and do the transplant. In September, I obliged as I turned twenty-one. It was determined that the final testing be done at the hospital when I came home for the Thanksgiving holidays. If all these tests went as expected, the kidney transplant would be scheduled for late January.

Suddenly, the whole situation became more real. What was once only the province of my mind, now was becoming a reality. What had also become real was that dialysis was going to be a painful struggle for Debbie. During the entire time my sister had been sick, she had many difficult moments. Yet I don't think anything upset her more than being on dialysis. One weekend when I was visiting from school, Debbie took me aside and told me about her experience on dialysis. She threatened never to go back.

It was a Friday night and I had just arrived home after a three-hour ride from school. I was starved. My timing was perfect though. My father had walked in from work just a few moments before me and dinner was just on its way to the table. After a quick hello, dinner began in earnest. The pot roast and potatoes and carrots were disappearing as quickly as my mom could refill my plate. I was so busy quenching my hunger that I didn't notice how quiet everyone was, especially Debbie. After dinner, my parents decided to go to a movie, and Debbie and I were just going to hang around the house.

It was not like my sister to show her emotions. She had become accustomed to stoically hiding her feelings. But after my parents left, she asked to talk to me. She seemed terribly vexed. I could see she was bravely attempting to hold back tears.

"What's the matter, Deb?"

"I can't do it anymore."

"What?"

"I can't stand it!"

"What are you talking about?"

"Dialysis. Larry, I don't know if Mommy told you, but it's horrible."

"No. No one told me anything."

"First I had to have surgery on my arm. They had to hook up an artery to a vein so that my blood return system could accommodate the dialysis machine. I know that machine is supposed to help me, but I hate it! They say that the first couple of times on the machine are the worst. I sure hope so because I don't know how I'm going to take being hooked up to that machine. I just can't stand it!

"I know I shouldn't complain. This machine keeps a lot of people alive. It's keeping me alive. But I have to lay on my back for five hours with needles sticking out of my arms. Sometimes the needles hurt so badly, my arms and back cramp up and I want to cry out to Mommy to help me. I feel so helpless!"

Her eyes were filled, almost brimming over the lids. Her nose turned red and she began sniffling. I thought she was about to cry; but instead, fighting back the tears, she pressed on.

"The worst part of it all is that I don't really feel any better when I'm finished with the machine. They say that you're supposed to feel good but I don't. I feel tired and dizzy. Larry, I'm not sure I can ever go back there." She began to cry. I put my arm around her. Shaking her head no as if to ward off the tears, she turned to me and resolutely said, "I feel terrified, but if I don't go back, I'll get sicker and die. I feel trapped."

Gently patting her on the back, I told Debbie to hang on. "You've got to go back. We'll be doing the transplant soon, and you won't ever have to go back to that machine." I felt so bad for her, but at that moment I was sure that things were about to turn. She just had to hang on a little longer. Crying seemed to make her feel better and she settled down. We ended up watching a movie on TV until my parents came home. That was the only time I remember seeing my sister cry over the entire time she was ill.

Everything was moving quickly and Thanksgiving came around too soon. I was not going to have the opportunity to savor the usual Thanksgiving feast. Before I knew it, I was checked into the hospital and on a table in some dark X-ray room having dye injected into my kidney from a tube that was inserted through an artery into my inner thigh. This test was called, appropriately enough, an arteriogram. It mapped out my kidney including the positions of renal veins and arteries for the purpose of deciding which kidney to take. When they injected the dye it burned like hell and I felt like jumping off the table. I clenched my fist and within fifteen to twenty seconds, it was over.

This was the highlight of a weekend filled with X-rays, blood tests, and all sorts of prodding and probing. One doctor after the other marched into my room, checking one bodily function or another. Without objection, I felt resigned to being put to the test. I must have passed with flying colors because the surgery was set for January 31.

It was a good thing, too. Debbie was still having a rough go of it on the dialysis machine. Her veins were collapsing which meant that she wouldn't last very much longer without a transplant. In fact, Debbie confided in me that if she had to continue dialysis, she would rather die. She seemed so desperate that I half-believed she meant it.

Debbie was seventeen and would turn eighteen in December. She had been sick since she was fourteen. Being in and out of school during that time was difficult for her. She missed out on so much. This is a time for young teenagers to explore and come of age. With all the promise and energy of youth sapped from her, she faced illness and death while most young girls were talking about boys, clothes, make-up, and parties.

While she had some good times during those years, Debbie's illness always lurked close by, a shadowy presence that clung to her, an essence that she couldn't shake. Occasionally, when she would go out with friends for a few laughs, she was able to take her mind off everything. Then she'd come home and a familiar shroud would envelop her. She was instantly transported back into a grim exile, marked by protracted suffering and a constant un-knowing of what medical malady the next day would bring.

Now, though, things were about to come to a head. The results were not guaranteed, far from it. This was not the per-fected procedure it became two decades later. Rather, it was on the cutting edge of new medical possibilities. Debbie was going to have a chance–to get off dialysis, have her energy back, and renew her life. My parents were going to have a chance to see their daughter grow up.

As for me, I only visualized a successful transplant. The thought of it not working didn't take root. Looking back at it now, I suppressed any self-congratulatory pats on the back that would rise to the surface. I thought of it as unseemly. A purely altruistic gift is given without asking for anything in return. Yet, deep down inside of me, there was a feeling that for the rest of my life, I would know that I made a difference in the lives of the people I loved. My parents' long nightmare of seeing their child deathly sick would come to an end. My sister's suffering and slow corro-sion would be transformed into a chance at life. She was going to have a chance to grow up, to become someone, to affect others, and to even change the world.

December rolled around and I had a heightened awareness of being very alone. It seemed that everyone around me was dealing with school, classes, and their social life. My life seemed in sus-pended animation. Long, cold walks through uncharted paths in the mountains, with only the sound of broken tree branches crack-ling underneath my feet, marked much of my time.

All thought had a singularity of purpose. I was preparing myself mentally and emotionally, undeniably bound for my desti-nation. I did my schoolwork diligently, but it mounted to little more than a minor distraction. I tenaciously held onto the feeling that this transplant was going to be a success. It was going to work. Debbie was going to be free, and my parents relieved.

January was too cold and snowy to walk. I huddled around the warm fireplace of a local bar and grill, sampling the soup of the day or having a glass of beer. In the corner, an old piano became a companion. As I played softly, I could feel my heart vibrating my emotions down into my fingertips and through the keys. Sometimes a friend would join me and we would talk; but the transplant seldom came up and if it did, only briefly. In my mind, though, it was an all-consuming mantra. I wasn't driven by any particular thought—just an ongoing, unyielding intention. It was an unwavering impulse generated from the core of my being, readying myself for the task at hand.

The week before the transplant, my parents were subdued and they seemed to shy away from any conversation dealing with what we were about to go through. Even my friends and Debbie's friends were at a loss as to how to deal with us.

January 30th finally arrived.

My mother, sister, and I found our way to the hospital admitting office. My father tried to avoid the ice my mother warned him about on his way back from parking our blue Buick. It was a long and cold walk from the parking lot to the hospital entrance. The admitting office was about ten yards from the front door, which didn't give my father much of an opportunity to warm up before he joined us. He looked frozen as he walked through the door.

We didn't know what we'd find after our two-hour ride to the Bronx. We were all happy that the hospital staff made us feel important. As it turned out, we were the hospital's first family doing a live donor kidney transplant. On one hand, we felt that we wouldn't be handled in a routine manner. Yet on the other hand, it meant that their experience was very limited.

After we were admitted and before we went upstairs to the "guest rooms," we found our way to the hospital cafeteria and got a bite to eat. We spent an hour there. My mother and father nursed two large mugs of coffee and shared a cheese Danish. Debbie picked at a slice of pizza and I quickly polished off a coffeecake. Before long, someone from hospital administration came to retrieve us. It was time to continue on the next leg of our medical odyssey.

Debbie and I were taken to different floors. My mom went with Debbie and my dad with me. It didn't seem right that they were splitting us up, but in a way it was symbolic. Ours were two distinct experiences. While this was happening to us as a family, it was also happening to us as individuals—four people bound together by this event, yet separated by the uniqueness of what was happening to each of us. We could all sympathize with each other but as in all things, the depth and power of our experiences are truly our own.

They settled me in a narrow room that didn't quite feel right. It was at the end of a long hall and it felt dark. A fresh coat of green paint made it seem somewhat undersized. There was a small window on the far side. I was disappointed that the bed near the window was occupied.

I met my roommate who was my father's age. We introduced ourselves. "Hi, I'm John Franklin, pleased to meet you." "The pleasure's all mine. I'm Ed Liebling and this is my son, Larry." He and my father exchanged additional pleasantries. I went over to my nightstand, opened the cabinet, and put away some history textbooks that I brought from school. My father and new roommate were still talking. Then John started to ask me a lot of questions. "Do you play chess? What programs do you watch on television? I saw you carrying some books, do you like to read?" Truthfully, he was annoying me. He talked too much, and I wanted to be alone with my thoughts. I had become very used to solitude. I wanted to get my bearings and had one thing on my mind—let's get this over with, let it work, and let me get out of here as fast as I can.

Afterward, my father said I should have been friendlier. Honestly, though, the man asked me a million questions when I needed to steel myself for what was to follow the next day. I am sure he was a nice man but socializing wasn't my top priority. I was starting to get nervous.

Before I knew it, they started the usual routine of taking body temperature and blood pressure. It seemed too early to be putting on the revealing hospital gown, but in an instant, my pants were gone and I was exposed. Feeling practically naked, I quickly put on a bathrobe and slippers.

My father and I decided to take a walk to see my mom and sister. We met them in Debbie's room. My mom seemed a bit nervous, but was trying to keep upbeat.

"Why did you change out of your street clothes?" she asked.

"They told me to," I answered. "They said that they had to start taking my blood pressure and temperature and it would be easier if I changed."

"They tried to get me to change also, but I decided since I'm going to have to wear this little hospital nightgown for quite some time, I'm not giving up my clothes yet." We all laughed, as Debbie held up the skimpy polka-dotted gown.

"Perhaps you should put it on anyway," my father said.

"Don't worry, Dad, everything's fine."

Debbie was talking optimistically and had an air of defiant bravery. The defiant part I understood because my sister was always strong willed and often defiant. The optimistic talk was a little unusual for her. More often than not, Debbie saw the difficulty in things and wasn't so ready to grasp a hoped for outcome.

I told Debbie and my mom about the annoying man with whom I was sharing a room. They both agreed almost simultaneously that maybe I should move to another room. My father said he wasn't that bad. Raising my eyes to the ceiling over his comment, I asked my mom to find out if after the surgery, I could have my room changed. She said she would see what she could do.

In a lighter moment, my mom and dad teased me about how long my hair was getting. The length of my hair had always been the subject of argument and debate ever since I was twelve. Now, at twenty-one, it was no longer the source of struggle between my parents and me, but it was still up for their review and comment.

My mom liked to playfully taunt me about my hair by retelling an amusing story that she used to emphasize how difficult it could be distinguishing between a boy with long hair and a girl.

"Larry, do you remember last summer when I had just come out of the supermarket?"

"Not that story again."

Over my mild objection and without hesitation, she began the recitation.

She had just finished her weekly visit to the neighborhood supermarket and was stowing her groceries in the car. After she loaded up the trunk to capacity, she was about to get in and drive away when she turned just in time to see a woman jump out of the way of a speeding car cutting through the parking lot. The woman immediately yelled, "Hey you, slow down."

She turned incredulously to my mom and asked, "Did you see

how crazy that girl was driving?" My mom said she most certainly did. She realized she recognized the car and that the "girl" inside looked very familiar. Adjusting her glasses, she realized that the girl was no girl at all, it was me. Not divulging my identity, she told the woman, "I know that girl's mother and believe me when I tell you, she's going to hear an earful."

When she got into her car, her mind raced. "How could he drive so fast? Wait until I see him." But as she drove away, she couldn't contain her amusement at how the woman thought I was a girl. Through her annoyance she let out a slight giggle. Arriving only seconds after me, she told me what happened. After promising not to drive so fast, I shook my head in amazement, wondering how anyone could mistake my bear-like, nearly six-foot frame for a girl.

"That's why you should get a haircut," my mom said.

"That's why I decided to grow a beard," I said, ending my mother's tale.

We all laughed again even though we had heard it several times before. That story always, as a matter of routine, led to making fun of the fact that my father appeared to have more hair on his mustache than his balding head.

As we made fun at my father's expense, a woman with strawberry hair leaned in, knocked at the open door, and excused herself for interrupting.

All too quickly, the hospital had sent someone to usher me back to my room. I was beginning to think that they were keeping track of my every move. The doctor that was doing my surgery wanted to discuss a few things with me. Debbie had her own team of surgeons who would attach my kidney to her once my team of doctors removed the kidney from me.

It was time to say good-bye. I kissed my mom and dad and

said goodbye to Debbie. She quickly admonished me, "Don't say good-bye, say goodnight." Good-bye sounded too permanent, like we weren't going to see each other ever again. Everyone felt weepy even as we were all trying to put up a brave front. My father decided to walk me back, though my mom felt she didn't want to leave Debbie alone. She promised to stop by my room before they left to go home.

The walk back was filled with small talk. My father launched into an ardent soliloquy about football and how lousy the Giants were this year. I was a thousand miles away, though, listening to the deepest part of me marking time, converging toward tomorrow. It turned out that the doctor who wanted to see me was called away. It didn't matter as it was getting late, and I knew my folks would have to leave soon.

It was about eight o'clock when my mom walked in. My dad and I were watching TV.

"It's time for us to go home," my mom said walking through the door. "Tomorrow is going to be a busy day and the transplant is set for 7:00 in the morning. Your father and I have to get up at 5:00 to get here in time."

"Goodnight, dear," my mom said as she kissed me.

"Remember we love you very much. Everything's going to go just fine. Tomorrow at this time, it will be all over."

"I know, Mom."

"I'll see you in recovery when it's all over," my father said as he kissed me on the cheek.

With that, they slowly turned around and headed for the door. When they reached the hallway, they looked back nervously, smiled, and waved. My mom blew a kiss and my father winked. I could hear their footsteps slowly fading, echoing down the hall.

They were gone. I was left with my talkative roommate who had thankfully fallen asleep watching TV. I guess he finally ran out of questions.

I sat back in my bed and thought to myself that tomorrow will be here soon. I felt a momentary calm, a pause between the spaces of everything that had led up to this moment and every-thing that was about to take place. Then I thought, it would be over soon. I visualized my parents standing next to each other with smiles on their faces. I could feel the warmth of their happiness.

I began to recall some of the things that happened to Debbie and myself while growing up–like the time that she drove my father's car on New Year's Eve. I laughed out loud remembering the frightful thought of possibly running into a bear during our great escape from sleep-away camp.

Then I had a funny daydream. Debbie and I were younger. It was autumn and she had tagged along with me on my way to play-ing football with some of the neighborhood kids. When we chose sides, as usual, they made me take my sister on my side. It was kind of stupid on their part because Debbie was actually a good player and held her own. But I guess they didn't want any kid sister on their side. The rest of my daydream amounted to one play–the final play of the game. We needed a touchdown to win. I was the quarterback and Debbie was going out for a pass. She started running down the field but she tripped and fell.

So I looked for someone else to pass the ball to but they were all covered. I was about to run with the ball when I saw that Debbie had gotten to her feet and was streaking down the field wide open. I threw the ball as far as I could. As I did, all the other kids disappeared from my dream. It seemed like the longest ball I had ever thrown and took an eternity to come down. Finally, though, the ball descended right into Debbie's arms. She held the ball tightly and ran over the goal line. We won. I ran downfield to my celebrating sister in the end zone, where we hugged and screamed out our victory.

Just then, a nurse came in to take my temperature and blood pressure and told me that Dr. Collins wanted to talk to me now. She escorted me to the doctor's office. As I walked down the hall, all I could think of were the smiles on my parents' faces and Debbie's touchdown celebration. The uneasy feeling that hovered over me earlier was gone. I felt a sense of calm.

Although Dr. Collins was six feet tall, he appeared slight. He was well dressed in a perfectly tailored navy blue suit and spoke in a proper English accent. I think he was actually South African. His full head of black hair was streaked with silver. Everything in his office was impeccably placed, from an engraved pen and pencil set sitting atop a leather desk blotter to a row of medical books neatly lined up on an oak credenza in the corner.

Sitting behind his desk, he was leaning back in a tall-backed brown chair. He invited me to sit down in a smaller chair across from him. We began to talk and he told me about the operation that was going to take place tomorrow.

While we had met briefly before, this was the first time that he and I were talking one on one. I didn't think much of the fact that we really didn't have that much contact until now because I was pretty well briefed on the procedure by the medical doctors who were overseeing the entire process. At least I thought I knew what was going to happen–that is, until he told me that they would have to cut away half of my lower right rib so that they could "harvest" my kidney more effectively. I was a little shocked. Maybe it was the word "harvest" or maybe it was the vision of cutting my rib, but it was then that I realized that physically, my body was going to change. I guess I was always picturing a successful end result and not the actual step-by-step physicality of it. It was at that moment that I understood that they were going to reach into the depths of my body, sever, and take a part of me.

Then he told me something that has stuck with me ever since. He said, "You're a very lucky young man to have the opportunity to do this for your sister." While I knew what I was about to do had a self-fulfillment component to it, I never quite looked at it as a golden opportunity.

I really thought that I was making a tremendous sacrifice. Was he trying to take me down a peg? I didn't think I was carrying myself with pride or arrogance. Perhaps he was just making sure that I realized that in giving this gift, I was also receiving a gift of a multi-faceted nature. Perhaps he was intimating that life gives us moments where we can step forward and change a result, and that by doing so we change ourselves.

To this day, I'm not really sure in what sense he meant it. At the time, I didn't pursue it with him. I just nodded my head. Yet when I recall those days, I remember his words and they continually prompt me to look deeper inside myself.

The rest of our conversation was short. As I got up to leave, he told me that another doctor would be in soon to do some necessary prep work. I said okay and he told me not to worry about tomorrow. He said that I was in a good hospital and they had an army of doctors and nurses working to make this a success.

When I returned, a nurse came in to tell me she had something to help me sleep. I had never taken a sleeping pill, and I told her it would not be necessary.

I hopped into the bed. One of the doctors who had previously conducted some tests on me came in. He told me that he was going to hook me up to the intravenous drip and put in a Foley catheter. I asked him what a catheter was. As he was explaining it to me, he unpacked a long tube and what looked like a hot water bottle from a shipping container.

As a kid, I had the usual cuts and bruises. There was never anything serious though, not even a broken bone. I could only hope that the insertion of the catheter was not the portent of pain and discomfort to come. Years later, when other people would recount a hospital surgery to me, I learned that their catheter was deployed while they were under a general anesthetic right before their surgery. I should have been so lucky! You could say what a pain in the neck that was, of course though, your description wouldn't be so accurate.

After the doctor left, the nurse came in with my sleeping pill. I no longer thought I wouldn't need it. The catheter had me jumping out of my skin!

Early the next morning, the fluorescent lights over my head woke me up. The nurse came in to take my temperature and blood pressure. I was drowsy and couldn't get my bearings. For a brief moment, I wasn't sure if I was dreaming or not. As the blood pressure cup tightened around my arm, I realized that morning had arrived and the process was about to begin. I asked the nurse if it was time to go. She said they would be calling for me momentarily. This was it! I felt the pull of fate fulfilling a promise initiated long ago. Events had taken on a life of their own, and I was playing my part in this family saga.

The nurse said she was going to give me a shot of something that would help me relax. She said it would make me woozy. By the time they came to get me, I was feeling quite comfortable. They put a cap over my head and covered my newly grown beard. Everything was happening quickly.

Within minutes, we left my room and headed to an elevator down the hall. Several people rode down with me. I guess they were doctors and nurses and I vaguely remember that they were gossiping about a hospital romance that sounded like a soap opera. Someone may have asked me a question as to how I was doing.

As the elevator doors opened, I saw Debbie. She had just arrived and also had a cap on her head. The two of us were on gurneys, and we took one look at each other and started to laugh. Maybe it was nervous tension being released, but it was nice to laugh with my sister. It had a bonding effect. At that moment, I felt closer to Debbie than I had ever since we were kids. Whatever frustrations there were between us simply melted away.

We waited there together for about five minutes, laughing and joking and generally exhibiting a high from the shot they had given us to "relax." Everyone who walked by smiled. We were obviously in good spirits.

There was nothing else to do now. There was no turning back. The course of our lives had intersected at the crossroads between life and death.

Soon the anesthesiologist would guide me to an unknown sleep. I knew in several hours I would awaken and in some defining way our fate would be determined. My sister would either be on a new journey pointed toward a brighter tomorrow or her life would be set adrift facing only the darkest possibilities.

What hand placed our lives in such an uncertain disposition? Only providence held the secret. But as I lay there waiting, anticipating, I knew I was ready. What I didn't know was that this drama would not cease to be with the end of the surgeon's skill that day. These moments would continue to echo through the rest of my days–a thread that weaves itself through the very fabric of my life.

They were ready for us. We waved to each other and said, "See you later," with smiles on our faces. As they wheeled us apart,

I remember whispering to myself, almost as if a prayer, "Debbie, catch the ball."

When I got into the operating room, they hoisted me onto the table quickly. The room looked smaller then I thought it would be. It seemed cold and had a stainless steel milieu. People were scurrying around. They started to hook me up to various instruments. Someone gently stretched out my arms, asked me if I was all right, and then told me to count down from ten to one. I anticipated further instructions, but by the time I reached the number eight, I was out.

9

❖ ❖ ❖ ❖

It couldn't have been easy for my parents that day. It's hard to comprehend what it must have been like for them. Certainly at the time, I couldn't appreciate the depth of anxiety they must have endured. As the surgical outcome of their two children remained out of their control, events had taken them down a path they never could have envisioned when they first began to raise their family. Their idyllic, suburban life–suddenly without warning–had disappeared.

They had to watch as their daughter slowly deteriorated over the course of four years, knowing all the time that only a miraculous turn of events could save her life. In spite of great odds, they had made it this far but now fate played with their hearts. The only good shot they had at her surviving was to put the life of their other healthy child at risk.

What a torturous knot to unravel! Their son agreed to go ahead with the transplant, but could they let him go through with it? What if the transplant is successful but something terrible happened to him? Could he die in surgery? What if the doctors made a mistake that injured him permanently? What if the transplant didn't work? They would be left with a mortally ill child and their best hope gone—while their son would have gone through all this for nothing. What would that mean for him psychologically? What if a catastrophe happened? What if a series of events occurred where both of them died? How could they ever live with themselves after that?

All the "what ifs" swirling, curving, bending the mind in search of the right road to take. Sometimes, though, no matter all the mindful turbulence, life propels us toward the inevitable. It's as if somewhere along the way, the only choice becomes to do nothing, ride the wave, fearful of the consequences by the shoreline, but hoping, praying to glide to safety unscathed.

Perhaps that's how it was for my parents. I was asked to donate my kidney to Debbie, took the necessary tests, was the perfect match, and agreed. My parents neither encouraged nor discouraged me. Now we were all ready to ride the wave.

The transplant was supposed to take six hours. As my parents sat in a small waiting room, an hour passed, then two. Someone sent word from the operating room that everything was going according to plan. The next few hours passed without a word. No one came to tell them what was going on. My parents decided to go to the coffee shop in the hope that the time would move faster.

When they returned, there still wasn't any message from the operating room. As six and a half hours turned to seven, my parents started to get very nervous. My father told my mom they probably didn't start exactly on time. As seven and a half hours turned to eight, my father jumped to his feet, began to pace, and facing my mother, he said, "If they hurt either one of those kids, I'll sue the pants off of 'em." My mom told him to calm down. "It won't do any good to talk that way."

My parents, now exhausted and emotionally drained from the nine hours, were beginning to fear the worst. Something must have gone terribly wrong for it to be taking so long.

Nine hours turned into ten and then eleven–and still there was no word from the doctors. What could be taking so long? Why won't they come and tell us what's going on? Someone should come and tell us what's happening. Do we dare ask? Finally, after twelve hours of a debilitating wait, the doctors called for my mom and dad.

Someone from the hospital came to get my parents.

"Mr. and Mrs. Liebling, the doctors need to see you down in the operating room area."

"Oh, that's not good, they only call you down if things are bad," said a woman also waiting for a loved one in surgery.

Unnerved by the long wait and the woman's comments, they were taken down the elevator to the doctors' lounge right outside the operating room where Debbie and I were. Haltingly, the doors squeaked open to an air of exhaustion. The doctors were waiting for them. Anxious, my mom and dad desperately waited for someone to tell them something. Dr. Everett, the head of Debbie's team, spoke first.

"Everything is all right. Both your son and your daughter are stable and the transplant went very well." A sense of relief immediately engulfed my parents. "We had a problem, though. Your son's kidney was in spasm and stopped working. We were prepared to wait a long time, which we obviously did, for it to start up again. Luckily it did, and we were able to continue with the transplant. We also had to realign the arteries in the kidney that we transplanted. All things considered, everything went very well. You two have been here for so long, you might as well go home, get some sleep, and come back fresh tomorrow."

"We want to see the kids before we leave," my mom said.

"Neither one of them has completely come around yet."

"We want to see them anyway."

They rushed into recovery to see my sister and me.

I had some vague feeling that someone was standing over me.

"Did they start yet?" I mumbled through an annoying clear plastic mask covering my face.

"Yes, it's over now," my parents said.

"Is Debbie okay?" I asked, but before I could hear an answer, I nodded out.

10

❖ ❖ ❖ ❖

"Help, someone help me." I awoke in terrible agony.

A nurse came over.

"Can I help you?"

"Yes, you can give me something for my side. Why does it hurt so much?"

She came back with a shot of painkiller. It seemed like an eternity; but within minutes, I felt relief. I had never experienced shooting pain like that before. I rarely thought about how much pain there would be after the surgery. I simply assumed there would be some. It seemed futile to worry about it because there wasn't any way that I could prepare for it.

As it turned out, I was completely surprised about how painful it turned out to be. However, I decided that I wanted to be brave and not whine. I thought it unseemly, not manly, and certainly I didn't want anyone thinking I was a complainer. It was my distinct expectation that pain was something you endured. So I was determined to take whatever painkiller I needed and not verbalize about the amount of pain I was in.

It was over but what had happened? Where was Debbie?

"Where is my sister?" I asked the nurse.

She pointed to the room next to me that was walled off in glass.

I started to turn to see where she was pointing to, but I couldn't move because I was in too much pain. I winced a bit and the nurse said, "Wait a minute. I'll help you shift over."

As she helped me, I saw my sister sitting up with a smile on her face. She had been awake for some time and waiting for me to come out of the anesthesia. She saw me struggling to turn around and she started to wave. With that, I knew everything had turned out well. The smile on my sister's face made me feel warm all over. I felt a brief moment of jubilation, but within a few minutes, I was sleeping again and allowing my body to start the process of healing.

The transplant was successfully completed in twelve hours. Debbie was in an isolation room to minimize the chance of being exposed to an infection. Infection would jeopardize her transplant and enhance the possibility of rejection.

With the surgical process over, all eyes were now on the question: How would Debbie's body respond? It was simply a given that the new kidney was viewed as a foreign object. Her immune system would immediately mobilize to reject the perceived invader. In order to combat this natural reaction, Debbie was given heavy doses of immuno-suppressant drugs. The catch, however, was that the drugs reduced her immunity to colds and other diseases, which could leave the kidney exposed to rejection. Her progress was to be measured first in hours, then in days.

Debbie would have to stay in isolation for a month until her body adjusted to the new kidney. Then, the doctors would slowly reduce the amount of immuno-suppressant drugs until they found a good balance. An equilibrium had to be established where she could leave the isolation room with the confidence that her body wasn't going to reject the kidney. Debbie would have to live the rest of her life on these drugs.

I was in the intensive care unit. They were keeping me there an extra day so that I could be next to my sister before they moved me to a regular room. I must say they tried to make me as comfortable as possible, but because my kidney had gone into a spasm, I was on the operating table for a long time in an odd position. The nurse told me that was why I was experiencing so much pain.

Soon I was transferred from intensive care to the floor I was on before the operation. I was thankful that it was a different room and a different roommate. My mom asked the head nurse if she thought I would need private nursing. She said the staff on the floor would take very good care of me and a private nurse would not be necessary. Indeed it wasn't.

One nurse in particular was determined that I made a full and speedy recovery. Her name was Maria. She was a tiny woman who wasn't much older than I was, but she mothered me and made sure that I was comfortable. Part of me was embarrassed that I needed help, but mostly I was grateful to have her. She was kind and encouraging and to this day, I remember her gentle touch.

My stay in the hospital lasted seven days. The first few days I mainly coped with my pain. With each ensuing day, I gained more and more strength. At first Maria helped me get out of bed, then get dressed; and finally she started me on laps around the hospital.

I didn't have too many visitors. A couple of kids from college came to see me. Of course, my mom and dad were there every day. They would shuttle back and forth between Debbie and me. I did receive a couple of congratulatory calls, a few cards, and a basket of fruit from my parents' best friends.

Before I knew it, I was strong enough to go home. Not so for my sister, whose stay would be at least another four to six weeks.

Anyone who wanted to see Debbie had to wear a cap, gown, and paper boots. We all looked pretty funny visiting her in the isolation get-up. One day, my sister laughed so hard at the way my father looked that she sent him out of the room because it hurt so much when she laughed. She was truly happy, although I think she was a little scared that her new kidney might reject.

My mom said that Debbie wanted to talk to me before I left to recuperate back home with my parents. I put on the mask and the funny paper boots and sat down in a chair next to her. We joked around for a bit and then Debbie said, "Thank you for giving me your kidney." But, then in a stunningly serious tone she added, "If you think this is going to change anything between us, you've got another thing coming."

My sister's rebellious nature came through loud and clear. Outwardly I laughed, but inside something hurt when she said it. I guess this was Debbie's way of letting me know that she wasn't going to feel like she owed me anything. Her response came as a surprise. It wasn't at all what I expected. All I wanted to hear and feel was a heartfelt thank you. I wanted her to put her arms around me and hug me so hard with appreciation. To me, I felt as if the whole world had changed.

I was also surprised and disappointed that no one really knew what to say to me after the transplant. Just like before the transplant, everyone's response, including my parents', was muted. While I failed to understand the silence before the operation, after the surgery, it puzzled me even more. Maybe my parents didn't know what to say. All I remember is longing for their approval. I always knew and felt that I had their love. Yet, after the transplant, I felt like there was something missing.

Sitting here now, in hindsight, I've come to realize that they must have been preoccupied with my sister's condition. Their mode of thinking must have changed almost instantaneously after the transplant. Before the surgery, they were concerned about Debbie's illness and the transplant outcome. As soon as the transplant was over, their concern must have switched to what happens if the kidney is rejected, what then? Any real celebration would have to be postponed indefinitely until we were assured of ultimate success. Of course, no one really knew when that would be.

Inwardly, I felt like I had acted with courage. In my mind, the transplant had been a success. I wanted to celebrate the relief that everything had gone so well. Yet, I seemed to be very much alone in that sentiment. I wondered what my parents thought. I was left to interpret the silence.

How we struggle to be liked, wanted, and recognized. Acceptance is a very fragile part of life. Most of us look for acceptance from many different sources. We look to our parents, our spouses, our siblings, our friends, and even strangers. We tend to ask others to accept us and confirm our own sense of who we are. We're inclined to look outside of ourselves to get the feeling that we're okay. All too often, we also look to others to validate that we are lovable. Right after the transplant, I think that's part of what I was looking for from my family.

Perhaps it was simply the child inside of me yelling, "Mom and Dad, look and see what a wonderful thing I've done!" Or maybe it was something inside of me proclaiming to the world, "I am important." I'm not really sure, but I know it was something that first made me feel hurt, then guilty, for wanting something in return for the gift I had given my sister. I think the muted response I received reinforced that feeling. I think I drove my hurt down deep into my soul. The guilt of wanting acknowledgement beyond what I received was impossible to leave on the surface of my mind. As much as I had a score of emotions before the transplant, it seemed that I was left with many unresolved feelings after the surgery.

Considering it now, I've lived with that unresolved ghost for the last twenty-two years. Maybe it influenced me more than I know, or more than I am willing to admit. Until this moment, I had only some vague feeling that I craved more attention from that episode. I suppose that if I let myself believe that, I would question my very motivation for donating the kidney to my sister in the first place. Was part of the reason I did it for the attention I would receive? Were my motives not as altruistic as I thought? I never let myself think that because if that was true, I couldn't even play the part of silent hero to myself. I never let myself think about it until now. All of a sudden, what was in the past seems to be surfacing unresolved. Could there be more?

11

❖ ❖ ❖ ❖

The day I left the hospital was dark and cloudy. The scent of snow was in the air even though it was not predicted in any of the weather reports. Coming home felt good, and I was relieved that my part was over. Yet, I shared my parents' concerns that Debbie's body would accept the new kidney.

The next few days I spent recuperating in my parents' home. It was a quiet time. My parents spent long hours visiting Debbie in the hospital. I remember looking out the window at a wintry landscape of bare trees, overcast skies, and the lawn dotted with patches of ice and snow. I recall watching a lone black bird, streaking across the sky bound for some unknown destination. He seemed to have lost his way. Somehow I felt like that bird because in the immediate aftermath of the transplant, I remember feeling somewhat confused and dazed.

I thought I'd feel a sense of contentment after the transplant, and I did briefly in a flash. It was just a glimpse of tranquility that glowed, then dimmed and quickly dissolved.

Instead, I could feel the power and uncertainty of change rush through my veins. I felt older. I felt as though part of me was disappearing. Maybe I was losing the flame of youthful aspirations. Or perhaps it was some sense of closure. Or maybe I was just confused and in need of renewal.

Whether I realized it or not, this last year of my life was focused on this event. It's funny because I really didn't think much about what I would do when the transplant was over. In a sense, it was like playing a role in movie. The characters are introduced, the plot lines drawn, everything converges toward a critical apex, then fades to black. When the movie is over and the popcorn and candy are all spent, everyone goes home. Well, I wasn't exactly sure where I was going. All I knew was that I had to get on with my life and find my path. But I also knew I felt lost.

Physically, it was still hard to straighten up without wincing. Yet after a few days at my parents' house, I decided it was time to go back to school. I had a few friends at school who welcomed me back without fanfare. The next day, I went back to classes; I felt that I couldn't afford to fall any further behind in my work. I had a hard time walking back and forth to class and discovered that I fatigued easily. Years later, I learned that recuperation from the type of surgery I had usually takes six weeks. I was obviously pushing it. I favored my right side, guarding it whenever I walked from one class to the other. I felt vulnerable.

The most dominant memory I have of that time, though, is that I wanted to talk to someone about what had just happened to me. As before the transplant, it was on rare occasion that I found someone willing to discuss it with me. Everyone seemed consumed by the same two things: schoolwork and their social life, and not necessarily in that order. While I had those same cravings, they paled in contrast to my need to share my experience. I felt like a stranger in a foreign land, exiled from a place that was more hospitable and congenial.

Back at home, everything was going well with Debbie. There were a couple of bumps in the road, but each one was weathered. She had a rejection episode that landed her back in the hospital for a few weeks. Concerned that things were about to unravel, I came down from school to visit her. I remember looking into my mom's eyes while I was suiting up to go into the isolation room. Silently she communicated to me, "Larry, do something." Of course I had already done all I could and felt rather helpless. Fortunately, the kidney didn't reject and Debbie never again had to go back to the hospital to fight a possible rejection.

Over the next few months, Debbie went for periodic testing to make sure that her new kidney was functioning properly. With each passing day, her health improved. Life returned to her cheeks again. Gone was the pasty ghost-like appearance of the past four years. Her face began to glow and blush. Her eyes sparkled, like a fire rekindled.

Soon, her visits to the doctors were cut back and then ended. Before anyone could realize, I graduated from college and Debbie graduated from high school and started college. My mother and father went back to their lives, too, but I think they were forever fearful that Debbie's kidney would reject.

12

❖ ❖ ❖ ❖

"Dad! Dad!" Josh said as he opened the sliding glass door.

"What, Josh?"

"Where'd Mom go?"

"She went to the grocery store to pick up a few things."

"Matt called and said all the kids are getting together at his house to hang out. Can you give me a ride over?"

"When do you have to go?"

"Matt said to come over in about forty-five minutes. Is that okay with you?

"That's not a problem."

"Okay, I'm going upstairs to get ready. Call me in forty-five minutes, okay?" he said as he went through the door, stopping briefly to pat Molly on the head.

Just then, Carolyn walked in with a bag of groceries in tow.

"You need a hand with that?" I asked her.

"No, I've got it."

"Are you still sitting outside? Still thinking about your sister?"

"I can't stop thinking about Debbie. Feelings and memories

that I haven't had in awhile are bubbling up to the surface."

"Are you sure you're all right?

"Don't worry, Carolyn, I'm fine."

"Can I do anything for you?"

"I just want to sit here for a while longer. If you don't mind, Josh is going to Matt's house in forty-five minutes. Can you give him a ride?"

"Of course, but are you sure you don't want to go? It might be a good idea to get out of the backyard for awhile." She tried to pry me from my retrospection.

"I'm really fine back here."

"All right, I'm going upstairs to put away the groceries."

"Don't forget to call your parents to see how they're doing today," she said.

"I'll give them a call a little later on this afternoon."

"Oh Molly, I bought a bone for you." She pulled out a chewy bone for Molly, tossed it to her, and then disappeared upstairs.

Wagging her tail as she inspected Carolyn's gift, Molly busily went to work first nibbling the edges, then all out gnawing. She devoured her bone completely, stopping only momentarily at the sound of another dog barking in the distance. Then she sniffed around for more and looked surprised when there was none.

Again I thought how lucky I was to be married to Carolyn.

How is it that some people have good marriages and happy lives and other people always have such a hard time? Why did my sister have to go through what she did?

I guess that's a question that everyone has asked at one time or another. I know there are all sorts of answers. Some people talk about reincarnation as a system that brings us back to earth as a laboratory for learning in all types of situations. Theoretically, that sounds plausible. In fact, I probably believe in it, but it doesn't answer the cries of people in real pain. That explanation soothes me when things are going well. When I see someone in pain because they've lost someone or they are hurt in some way, it loses some of its potency. Maybe it is a question that is never meant to be understood with certainty. Perhaps it is a measure of my faith, but for me it remains unresolved.

As a father of a thirteen-year-old boy, I want him to have the very best of life. I don't want him to struggle and feel the pain that I know life can often dish out. Like all parents, I pray for his happiness and that he will have the opportunity to give something back to the world. When you are a part of gifting to the world another soul, you want that soul to take flight and soar.

When I gave my sister a kidney, I felt very much the same way. I wanted the best for her. I wanted her to find happiness and joy and to feel life renewed. I'm not sure, however, that it was that way for her.

Right from the beginning of the post-transplant era, her travail was not at an end; only the chapter had changed. Even though the transplant had gone well and she was feeling much better, the medication she was taking had some hard-to-live-with side effects. Her appetite grew exponentially. She said, "If it wasn't tied down, I'd eat it." She immediately blew up, her weight swelling her face well beyond the norm. She would walk into a room and you could see in people's faces the question, "What the hell happened to you?"

The truth was that no one could give Debbie any real idea of the long-term side effects of the drugs. She complained of feeling spacey all the time. She knew she needed the drugs to stay alive, but she also knew she was taking strong drugs that probably would have some adverse effects on her physically. While these powerful drugs were essential to her survival, they nevertheless came along with an unknown and nameless uncertainty.

Other issues also surfaced. Before the transplant, the central concern was Debbie's illness. After the transplant, the central concern was how long it would last. What wasn't so apparent was how the transplant was going to change everyone's lifestyle. Now Debbie had to be careful not to enter into situations where someone might have a cold or any other sickness—no matter how common or seemingly harmless. For Debbie, no germ was innocuous. Her immune system was suppressed to prevent the new kidney from rejecting. This left her immune system compromised. It also meant that friends and relatives couldn't visit unless we were assured they were healthy. We had to be careful not to get sick, too.

Whether it was before the transplant or after, the same core issue existed. Our awareness of life's fragile nature was heightened. That awareness became a way of life.

After awhile, some things started to settle into a "normal" state of being. Happily, the doctors were able to slowly reduce some of the medication Debbie was taking. Her swelling went down, and she felt a little less spaced out. It was a good thing, too, because the side effects made her social life difficult.

I had hoped that with the transplant, all the hurt of the past few years would go away, and everyone would live happily ever after. I was optimistic that the joy of life before Debbie's illness would return, and the memories of watching my sister deteriorate and seeing my parents despondent would be gone forever.

For me, life needed sorting out, but for Debbie there was a whole new set of circumstances to navigate. She tried hard to put her life together. She went to college, got good grades, and eventually received her doctorate in psychology. She liked the university atmosphere and felt very safe and secure. She enjoyed the challenge of discussing different philosophies with professors and students. Debbie studied long hours, driving herself endlessly to reach her goals. Once she told my mother that since her body betrayed her, she was determined to use her brains. It was especially gratifying to all of us to see her get her doctoral degree in psychology.

She also taught herself how to play the guitar and would spend endless hours learning all kinds of music, from rock to folk to rhythm and blues. She learned about photography, bought a camera, and specifically loved to photograph nature.

Sadly, after she graduated and as Debbie's life developed, I wasn't sure whether she was happy. Sometimes she'd be up and vibrant, yet at other times–too many times–she appeared unhappy about something.

She had high career expectations and was often disappointed. Unfortunately, she ended up bouncing around from one job to another. She would work at one place for awhile, feel good about it, but then sour. She often thought that the people she worked for were disorganized or lacked professionalism. Sometimes work was boring and monotonous. At other times, she complained about being overworked, under-appreciated, and underpaid.

While the workplace often left her discouraged and disillusioned, her social life was even more challenging. There was one difficult relationship after the other. She'd go out with someone and imbue that person with the most admirable qualities only to soon become greatly disappointed. On the other hand, several times she ended relationships because the person she was seeing was getting too serious and wanted to get married. From the outside looking in, I got the feeling that Debbie was always searching for a happiness that eluded her. I could feel her disappointment and I felt frustrated for her.

Perhaps happiness eludes too many of us. Maybe it is in our nature to always be longing for something. I sometimes wonder if we are ever satisfied with who we are and what we have. Maybe some of us are better than others at hiding our yearnings. Or maybe our culture doesn't teach us how to feel secure in our appearance, our status, or our sexuality. It seems to me that we are bombarded with continual images that flash before us and are impossible to fulfill.

In the end, do we betray our lives by listening to too many external messages instead of listening to our own heart's passion? I am not sure. But if we are lucky, after we muddle through all the voices we hear, we come to realize that we have an internal compass. It is a voice that tells us to choose. It's a call from deep inside us that softly utters who we are and why we're here. It tells us that we have a significant role to play as part of a greater whole. It tells us to choose to create joy, to recognize it, and to be grateful once it materializes.

Unfortunately, as my sister searched to discover who she was, I think she was often too hard on herself. I even wonder sometimes if she judged herself unworthy of happiness. Whatever it was, too often, she gave me the impression that she didn't relish life as I had hoped. She seemed lonely. At times, she'd find a way to sabotage her own best interest. All too often, she left herself needing to pick up the pieces in search of a fresh start. Years after the transplant, Debbie was physically in great shape but still struggling to be happy. She was still struggling to find her role. But my sister was a determined fighter. She never gave up and continued the search to discover herself.

As a result of the transplant, Debbie and I did develop a special relationship. Yet it wasn't as I expected it to be. There wasn't a transformation that moved Debbie and I especially closer to each other. Rather, because of the unique experience the two of us shared, we became linked by this event that intersected our lives. It was a distinct affinity we shared that no one else we knew had experienced. Yet, we operated on two different wavelengths as we had before the transplant. As has often been cited, two siblings raised by the same parents can be so different and so we were. Yet at the same time, there was something between us, something that tied us together, even if we didn't completely understand its complexity.

Year after year passed. On January 31st, we'd celebrate as another milestone passed and Debbie's kidney didn't reject. At some point, I stopped thinking that it would. Yet as we marked each anniversary, I waited and expected that special thank you from my sister that the year before she neglected to say. I often wondered if perhaps my sister, on some level, knew that I wanted her thanks. Maybe it was a power she held over me. After all, I was her older brother and sibling rivalry runs very deep.

Soon, however, I stopped expecting it. Maybe, too, over the years, I became used to being unacknowledged. Maybe I even slipped into the part, a role that made me an unacknowledged hero, a silent martyr in a solitude that became familiar, like a well-worn suit that hangs effortlessly, draping and hugging in all the right places. Yet somewhere inside, I still harbored a spark of hope that the unexpected would happen. Sometimes I would feel as if she was about to say something to me. But then inexplicably the moment was gone, only an aberration.

Sitting here now and looking back, I suspect that I harbored feelings of resentment. A sort of silent festering under the surface, a subtle bitterness, which over time must have seeped into the fabric of my mind–and probably got in the way of our relationship.

Yet in spite of this quiet unnoticed invader, which now surfaces to stab at my conscious, Debbie and I were bound forever, to this event, and to each other.

While the transplant karmically connected us, our lives took two very different paths.

Life seemed to favor me. While I had my fair share of adversity, Debbie seemed to be going through life with 50-pound weights attached to her ankles. While my problems found resolution, Debbie's difficulties always seemed to become compounded. One thing was certain; the road I traveled brought me great joy. It was the kind of happiness that comes unannounced. My dreams were being fulfilled. I got married, bought a house, and had a child. By comparison, it seems to me that Debbie's dreams were never really able to take off in flight. That is not to say that Debbie was always unhappy. There were laughs and good feelings but at critical points in time, and in significant areas of her life, events almost always conspired to hold her down. I often wondered why.

Part Two:
Lunchtime
Same Day
September 1, 1996

❖ ❖ ❖ ❖

13

❖ ❖ ❖ ❖

"Larry, I'm taking Joshua over to Matt's house. Do you want anything while I'm out? It'll be lunchtime soon. Should I pick up something?" Carolyn called to me.

"Why don't you stop at the deli for some sandwiches for us?"

"Sure. What do you want?"

"I'll take a turkey sandwich on rye with some Russian dressing, and see if they'll toss in an extra pickle."

"Okay, but I might be a while. I have a couple of stops to make," she said.

"Fine, that's fine, I'll see you in a while," I responded.

Josh yelled, "See you later, Dad." Carolyn added, "I'll be back shortly with lunch." Then in unison they both said, "Good-bye, Molly."

Molly stood up as Josh and Carolyn exited the front door. I think the dog was getting a little antsy sitting with me all morning long. She looked at me as if to say, "Where are they going?" but then became distracted by a flock of Canadian geese flying overhead. I watched as she followed them glide across the sky. I couldn't help wonder what she was thinking. Perhaps she wondered how they do that. Me too, Molly, I said softly aloud.

The morning sun that had glistened and glimmered through the leaves and tree branches soon gave way to noon. Everything gushed and erupted yellow and gold. I took a deep breath and could feel myself once again drifting down memory's corridor.

Like all parents, mine wanted to see their children happily married. I guess it's like getting a diploma—you did a good enough job as a parent that another human being would be interested in living with your child.

My parents were no different. Debbie was still attending graduate school so their marriage expectations for her weren't quite in high gear, but nonetheless, they worried if someone would marry her because of the transplant. I was a different story. I was out of school, working, and definitely a prime candidate for the heavy push toward marital bliss. Though it took awhile, I acceded to their wishes.

Carolyn and I met five years after the transplant.

I met Carolyn on the rebound. I know conventional wisdom says that meeting people after they've been in a long-term relationship never works out. Even the pop psychologists on talk radio say it isn't the wisest thing to do. Well, in our case, conventional wisdom and talk radio psychologists couldn't be more wrong.

It was the classic story of marrying the girl next door—well, not exactly. I had just moved into a converted apartment. Irene, my new landlady, had renovated the upstairs of her waterfront home into an apartment. The view outside Irene's upstairs window sold me immediately. Even though it was winter, the icy blue water held me spellbound. In the day, the sunlight dashed between the snapping whitecaps. It had an enchanting radiance and at night, the moonlight shimmered across the open bay and bleached out to sea. There was a private outside stairway entrance that led to a deck. I envisioned having summer time barbecues, sipping on a glass of wine, and watching the blaze of a summer's day be soothed by the onset of the evening sky.

Of course, as I was to find out, it also had its drawbacks. The rooms were cold and drafty. It was a considerably colder winter then usual. The snow had come earlier and more often than the previous year. The frigid wind blowing off the bay forced me to get a space heater. There was no remedy to the shower, though. The hot water lasted about ten seconds. When I asked Irene about it, she told me to wash the important parts. I told her I would have to go into Olympic training to complete the task in the allotted time.

I was pretty excited with my new apartment, warts and all. But I was also recovering from a broken romance. I was engaged to Laurie, a girl that lived in my old neighborhood. It ended abruptly when she said that things weren't going to work out. Something deep inside me knew that she wasn't right for me either; but somehow when someone wants to break up with you, suddenly he or she becomes the one and only person you can't live without.

So I was recovering from the breakup when I moved into Irene's. I wasn't there longer than three days when, upon my arrival home from work, I found Irene roaming around my apartment giving a tour of the place to these two women.

"Larry, I was just showing Carol and Carolyn the apartment. Carolyn lives right across the street, and her friend from work is visiting her," she tried to explain.

"That's nice, Irene. Be sure to show them the view," I said.

With that, they took a hasty look out the window and quickly left. They must have been embarrassed. Anyway, after they left, Irene was peppering me with questions about what I thought of

Carolyn.

"She's nice, isn't she? Would you like her phone number?"

Ever since I was a youngster, I knew I wanted to share my life with someone. I wanted someone who I could talk to and who could talk to me. Someone to take the journey with me. Someone to laugh with me. Someone with whom to have a family. Someone who would hug me when life got frightening and someone who I would comfort and embrace, too. Together we would chase away the darkness when things got too rough. I didn't want just anybody. I wanted to be married, but I wanted more than that–I wanted a soulmate. What's more, I thought that's the way it should be.

The problem was that I really hadn't come close to that ideal. It always ended up that I'd go out with someone for a while and one of us would realize that it wasn't going to work out. I started dating just to have a good time, thinking that if I wasn't looking for a relationship, I would find one. That is more "conventional wisdom." In the back of my mind, I was always on the lookout for the right person.

"Well, do you want her number? She's really very nice, and I think you two might hit it off," Irene said.

Well, in fact, she was pretty and I figured it wouldn't hurt me to go out on a date. So I thanked Irene and took her number.

It took me a week to get up enough nerve to ask her out. I called her on the following Tuesday for a date on Saturday. I wanted to be proper and all that. Even after she said yes, I was unsure that it was the right thing to do. Was I over Laurie? In some ways, I felt like I was cheating on that relationship. But that relationship was over and the sooner I realized that, the better.

I picked up Carolyn promptly at seven. We decided on a quiet seafood restaurant located on the water's edge. There's a certain energy and excitement that comes from being young and going out on a first date, and it was in evidence as we walked in and sat down. Soft candlelight warmed the night and eased our way.

At first, I was doing a lot of talking. I think that was partly because I had a lot on my mind and partly because I was afraid of any silence. I found it easy to talk to her. She was a good listener. I felt, though, that I was monopolizing the conversation so I asked Carolyn about herself. I found out that she was an accomplished conversationalist, more than willing to review her life's history.

As the candle melted, a soft light darted between us. A gentle rain danced on the rooftop and the hours passed. Table after table emptied, yet Carolyn and I still hadn't run out of conversation. I was pretty happy with the way the evening was going. A pleasing dinner was over. The coffeepot that had warmed by the tableside was now empty. Before we knew it, we were on our way home.

It's always awkward at the end of a first date. I had a good time and I thought she did, too. So I figured that a goodnight kiss was in order. I was hoping I had gauged the situation properly. As it turned out I did, because she was receptive to my romantic gesture.

After our kiss, I told her I'd call her and we said good-night. She disappeared behind the front door of 311 Riviera Drive South, taking her warm, rich smile with her.

I walked across the street. Pretty successful, I thought, scrambling up the steps two at a time. As I reached the front door, I lit up inside. Maybe this could be something.

By the time I entered my darkened apartment, I became cautious and said aloud, "Let's just take it one step at a time."

I called her again early in the week for a date on Saturday. This time we went to the movies. Unfortunately, I picked a real loser of a movie, but it didn't seem to matter. After the movie, we braved the cold and went for hot fudge sundaes. Even though this was only our second date, it felt like we had known each other for a long time.

It turned out that Carolyn was also getting over a long-term relationship. She was left a bit confused by her experience, but enough time had gone by that she was able to regain her equilibrium and was ready to start dating again.

As time went on, we went out more and more. We started to go out for dinner in the middle of the week and we spent all weekend together. While it was apparent to both of us that we were drawn to each other, we were also somewhat wary. Fresh from the wound of the previous relationship, I was very concerned about the future. Carolyn, too, was hesitant. She wanted to make sure that I was truly over my past relationship with Laurie.

Carolyn was scheduled to go away on vacation for a week to visit her parents in Florida. She felt the time away from each other would give us an opportunity to reflect on our relationship. We joked that when she came back, I could give some sort of sign as to how I felt about us. She said that if I wanted to continue the relationship, I should hang a flag out of the window where she could see it and she'd know that the romance was on. We laughed and kissed each other good-bye. I wished her a safe trip and off she went.

At first, the week went by as any other. Soon, however, I found myself constantly thinking about us and realized that we really had something. I didn't know where it would lead, but I knew that I wanted to continue seeing Carolyn, notwithstanding my apprehension about the future.

It was a cold clear Saturday night and I was alone in my apartment. I had just finished dinner and was listening to music when I suddenly remembered the flag. Anxious not to lose the opportunity to display my feelings in a humorous way, I immediately used my creative prowess to fashion a homemade flag out of a metal clothes hanger and white freezer paper from the kitchen cabinet. I took out the scotch tape from my utility drawer and put together the welcome home sign. I hung it out by the porch so she could see it from across the street and waited for her to come home.

That evening, around 7:30, I heard someone hurriedly climbing the stairs. There was a knock at the door. It was Carolyn with a smile on her face from ear to ear. "I saw your flag and came right over."

"I missed you," I told her as we embraced. With that, Carolyn and I had turned the corner in our relationship. Bonds that have lasted and strengthened over the last eighteen years found their origins with that moment.

As the winter's cold gave way to the soft warm breezes of spring, our days were filled with love's embrace and tender affections. We introduced each other to friends and relatives. We had long talks about everything and anything. We discussed and reflected about politics and religion and money and God. We revealed our feelings about having children; we talked about work and cars and the weather. We delighted in each other; and without even realizing it, we were creating a vision together.

We probed our worries and hidden concerns and even explored our fears. I told her all about Debbie and the transplant. She listened intently, wanting to know about everything. She gave me the opportunity to talk about every aspect of the transplant. I told her things I never was able to express to anyone else. Not only did she want to know every detail of what took place, but she also wanted to know how I felt about everything.

We seemed to be on a course to get married. A bond between us was forming that would fuse our lives together as we faced the future.

It seemed as if destiny had brought us together. Through the grace of God, our lives were about to move beyond what either of us had ever known. Events transpired to draw us closer.

One morning, I awoke to a knock on the door. I put on a robe and ran to answer it. It was Irene. She had something important to tell me.

"I wanted you to know that I'm not going to be around this summer."

"Don't worry, Irene, I'll look after everything for you."

"Well, that's what I wanted to talk to you about. I rented out the rest of the house to a family who will look after things. You don't have to worry, though, you can still stay upstairs."

"That sounds good to me. When will they be moving in?"

"Next week."

Over the next few days, I could hear Irene downstairs cleaning and preparing the house for the new tenants. I wondered what they'd be like. In a way, I was looking forward to new neighbors. Perhaps we could be friends. I thought that inviting them to dinner would be a real neighborly thing to do. My homemade lasagna always went over well. Of course I had to consider that perhaps they would prefer to just keep to themselves, which was all right too.

A week passed and a small moving van pulled into the driveway. It was followed by a white Volvo station wagon. Out stepped a young woman, two small children, a girl and a boy, and a huge dog with a menacing disposition.

Irene stepped out to meet them and Carolyn and I walked over from across the street to say hello. We had been sitting on

Carolyn's front steps admiring the morning and deciding what we were going to do on this wonderful spring day.

Irene introduced us to my new housemates. Jackie Thomas was slender and tall. Her blonde hair curled flawlessly down the front of her strapless white sundress. I extended my hand and said, "It's nice to meet you, you're going to love it here. The view is so wonderful." I was met with a less than enthusiastic handshake and an obligatory "Nice to meet you, too." She wasn't very friendly. When I tried to pet the dog, she told me to be careful because he was a guard dog and not to be trifled with. Just then, Irene's boyfriend, Roger, came to pick her up and off they went on a traveling summer vacation.

An eerie feeling came over me. My spring of love and merriment was about to take a detour. It was my distinct impression that this woman didn't like that I was in the house living upstairs.

It didn't take long for my feelings to be borne out. The next morning, I quickly got dressed, rushed through a cup of coffee, and off I went to meet Carolyn at her house. We made plans to take a walk on the beach. As I stepped out onto the deck, I took a deep breath. The morning air was infused with a salty mist. Huge, pearl white clouds gracefully swept across a cooling blue sky. Looking out to sea, I watched sailboats gliding atop the turquoise and navy blue waters of the Great South Bay.

Down the stairs I went, filled with the energy of a new day. I jumped off the last step and was completely startled when I was met at the foot of the stairs by a snarling, chained akita. When I say chained, it looked like he was going to snap out of that tether at any moment. To avoid being snapped at, I jumped off to the side. Without catching a breath, I ran across the street to Carolyn's house. My mind was racing. Something was going to have to change. I wasn't going to live with that.

Arriving at Carolyn's house was like reaching "home base." She told me to calm down and that she was certain that Jackie would make sure that the dog was tied up properly and in a place that wouldn't be so threatening.

After pacing around, worrying about what I was going to do for ten minutes, I decided that Carolyn was right. Jackie probably didn't realize that she had the dog so close to my entrance. So I decided to call her right away and resolve the situation as soon as possible so that Carolyn and I could go back to enjoying the day. Much to my surprise, Jackie was completely hostile. She told me that the akita was her protection. Her husband was often gone and she wasn't about to restrain the dog in any way. In fact, it was her intention to make sure that the whole neighborhood knew that Miko was big, bad, and ready.

I got pretty upset. I wasn't sure what I could do. Irene had left a number where she could be reached in case of an emergency. She was staying with her daughter in New Jersey for a few days before she officially started her vacation. So I called, but for the second time in one day, I was completely shocked at someone's reaction. Irene said that Jackie had the right to have the dog tied up anyway she wanted to. I told Irene, "You won't be too happy if the dog breaks through the chain and goes after a kid or something."

Irene told me that she thought I was being unreasonable and that wasn't going to happen. Then I told her that I would have to move if she didn't do something about the dog. I guess I miscalculated again. I forgot that I was renting out an upstairs apartment and not the rest of the house. Irene saw bigger dollar signs with Jackie and the dog rather than with me because she said that if I wanted to leave, that's my choice.

Well, I was in a little bit of turmoil. I don't like moving. It's not that I had a lot of stuff to pack. It's just that it took me a little while to find a place where I felt comfortable. I had canvassed many different apartments before I settled in at Irene's. I was also disappointed because I had endured the cold winter in that apartment and was looking forward to the warmth of the summer's sun by the bay.

Carolyn's mom and dad, Betty and Kal, were snowbirds. That's what they call people in Florida who spend the winter months in the "orange state" and fly back up north for the spring and summer. They had arrived back from Florida just in time to get in on finding a solution to my dog-initiated plight. They told me not to worry, that they had a lot of friends in the area that had rooms for rent, and finding a new place wouldn't be that hard.

So Carolyn and I went around to a couple of her mom's friends, but I didn't see a place that really interested me. Every apartment we saw was either too small, too dark, had no view, or just didn't feel right. I was getting pretty upset because I was real tired of avoiding Miko, who seemed to be turning my life upside down.

Yet even the dog couldn't take the shine out of the relationship that was developing between Carolyn and me. Everything was happening rather quickly. Things had a magical feel to them. We were on the same wavelength. But more than that, life had a sheen to it that I never experienced before. Carolyn and I were falling in love. I began to seriously think about asking Carolyn to get married. I wanted to be careful, though, because everything seemed to be going so fast.

Then one morning, after successfully dodging Miko, I was sitting in my office at work, when I thought to myself that all the pieces were coming together. Carolyn and I just seemed to fit right. Thinking about us warmed me inside. There was an aura that surrounded us that conveyed to the world and ourselves "destined to be." I could avoid it for a little while if I wanted to, but I didn't even want to.

That night, I came home and quickly went over to Carolyn's, who had gotten home from work a half hour before me. I was pretty excited about asking her, partly because I felt she wanted it too.

Looking back at it now, I suppose I could have been more romantic, but instead I went for the quick strike. Carolyn answered the door and kissed me hello. I could hardly contain myself. I felt like bursting out the news right then and there.

"What do you want to do for dinner?" she asked.

"Oh, I don't care. Should we go out?"

"Okay, where do you want to go?"

"How about the Oaktree Cafe?"

"Okay, I'll be right back. I just want to get a sweater."

"Where are your parents?" I asked.

"They went to meet Jennie and Manny at Santosha for dinner."

"Carolyn, before we go, I have a couple of things I want to talk to you about.

"Okay. We can sit in the living room."

I was getting excited to tell her. I could tell that she knew something was up. She probably knew what I was up to the minute I walked in the front door. We quickly sat down, and after the briefest pause I asked her:

"Do you want to get married?"

"Yes," she said with excitement.

There was no equivocation. The celebration was on. Carolyn immediately went to the phone to call everyone and anyone. She was on cloud nine and so was I. It was as if a great dam had burst.

The two of us had waited for this moment all our lives and it had finally arrived. We decided to get married in the fall. As we bathed in the glory of the moment, the simple joy we felt left us tingling.

Carolyn's mom and dad finally came home. The minute they opened the door, Carolyn yelled out that we were getting married. Her dad headed for the closet and pulled out a bottle of champagne. Her mother went down the hall toward the bedroom. She came out with a gold chain that was a family heirloom she planned to give to Carolyn on the day she got engaged.

There we partied for an hour until I realized we should go over to tell my parents. While it was late, I couldn't think of not going over to tell them. My father was sleeping and my mother was sitting in the kitchen having a late-night snack. My sister, who was still living at home, knew immediately the reason why we were there so late. My sister always worried about me and when I would get married. I think she worried that no one would want me because I had only one kidney.

So we partied some more with my folks and then took off to go back home. When I dropped Carolyn off, her mother was still up and told me that there was no sense in finding an apartment now. She said that they had a spare room I could use until we got married. It was left empty when Carolyn's brother, Jerry, moved to the city to continue his dream of becoming a standup comedian.

So within the span of a week, I had gone from being a bachelor in a bay side apartment, to a young man looking to run away from a mad dog, to a guy that was going to settle down and get married.

I had found what I was looking for. I had found someone I could love with all my heart and someone who would love me with all her heart. For the next four months, we prepared for a wedding, schemed about the future, bought a house, and had a lot of fun doing it.

I lived with Carolyn and her parents until October 20th. The day before our wedding, I went back to my parents' house for one more night and on October 21, 1979, we were married. All our friends and family danced and celebrated into the evening. The good wishes and joy that everyone had for us has remained within our hearts ever since.

Here it is nineteen years later. It's pretty hard to believe but with each passing year, I love my wife more and more. As we both suspected, we grow closer and closer each day. Sharing a journey that is enriched by our partnership, surely God has watched over us. Thank goodness that Carolyn didn't listen to any radio talk show psychologist. I guess you can catch someone on the rebound successfully.

Of course, my parents and Debbie were overjoyed. Carolyn asked Debbie to be her maid of honor. Carolyn's brother, Jerry, was my best man. Over the years, our two families have grown extremely close. Our marriage was more than just the marriage of two people. It was the marriage of two families. We became an extended family. Carolyn's mother, father, and brother became my concern and joy, as did my mother, father, and sister become hers.

14

❖ ❖ ❖ ❖

"Larry, I'm back. I brought some sandwiches. Do you want to eat out here or do you want to come upstairs and eat in the kitchen?" Carolyn asked, opening the door to the backyard.

"The weather is perfect for a backyard picnic lunch."

"Sounds good to me!"

"How are you doing? What have you been thinking about?" she asked as we began to eat lunch.

"Most of the morning, I was thinking about Debbie and the transplant. I've been recounting the whole history and trying to get in touch with my feelings," I said.

"And what kind of things have you thought about? Can I help you sort it out?" she asked.

"It almost seems like, now I'm looking at the past with different eyes. My memories are filtered through the lens of the present moment. The past seems to be teaching me new lessons about myself. With everything that has happened to Debbie this past year, I've been reviewing the circumstances surrounding the transplant. I've been rethinking everything, questioning and doubting.

I think I have a tendency to be hard on myself and maybe even too hard on Debbie and my parents. Yet that event continues to gnaw at me."

"Larry, I know the last year hasn't been easy. You would have to expect that issues would resurface. Sometimes the present jars a past moment from the cobwebs and holds a key to something that truly is meant for you to take a good, hard look at," she said. "It could also be that something that is happening now gives resolution to a memory and it comes out to claim completion. This is an important part of a process. If you try to suppress your feelings because it's hard to look at, it will only come back at some later date."

"You're right. I sense there are answers stored somewhere inside me. It's like these subconscious impulses are there waiting to be discovered. Lessons calling out to be learned."

"I think that happens to all of us. I think we suppress our feelings, without allowing them to find a healthy outlet, and that only hurts us and our own best interest." After a few moments of silence, she continued, "Try not to be too hard on yourself. Even though I agree with you that it's important to hash things out, it's also essential that you find a balance. Growth is important, too, but so is recognizing where you are now. Never forget how lucky we are to have each other and Josh," she said.

"I can never forget that. I thank God everyday for the life we've built," I said.

"Me too," she responded.

We sat for a moment or two. Then Carolyn asked, "Do you want to take a walk or something? The exercise will do you good."

"No. I'm going to sit here for a little while longer. Why don't you take Molly for a walk if you feel like getting some exercise?"

"Molly, you want to go for a walk with me?" Carolyn asked,

waiting for a response. I half expected Molly to say "No thanks. I'm going to stay here with him. I think he needs my company."

But she didn't. Instead, she looked at me and I said, "Go ahead, girl, take a walk." She wagged her tail and then put her head into my lap. She seemed to want to stay, and it was true that I was enjoying her company anyway.

"I guess I'll just have to go on my own." Carolyn said. "Better yet, I think I'll go to the shoe store. I've been looking for a pair of shoes for the winter. I'll only be gone for an hour or so."

"That'll be fine. I'll still be here in the back," I said.

"You sure you don't want to go for a walk? Maybe you want to go for a ride with me to the shoe store?" she asked.

"Me. You must be kidding! No way," I said.

"I didn't think so. I just thought I'd ask. I shouldn't be too long. Keep an ear open for the telephone. Josh might call. He wasn't sure when he was coming home," she said.

"If you end up at the mall, bring me one of those oven-baked salted pretzels they sell at that pretzel hut," I said.

"Okay, I'll see you soon."

Carolyn dashed out the front door. Lunch was over quickly. I don't even remember what I ate. Oh, a turkey sandwich. Anyway, I was glad to have her company. She has always been there for me to talk to. It seems like we've always been together. Our marriage seems to flow easily. I think that's because we are willing to talk to each other about anything. We don't hide our feelings. That is not to say that we haven't been presented with difficult moments.

Certainly we've had our difficulties, but we seem to be able to see our grace through the rough times. Even the circumstances surrounding Joshua's birth were not easy. Yet through those arduous and difficult days, we were able to see the hand of divine providence.

It's hard to believe that Joshua is thirteen years old now. Carolyn and I adore him. He's our only child. Josh is just the greatest kid ever, and I tell him all the time. I don't want you to think I spoil him...well, I guess I do.

He is growing so fast, too fast. It's a daunting task to keep up with his questions. He's smart, loving, and has a great sense of humor. There's also the gleam of a mischief-maker in his eyes. And eighth grade homework has us arguing more than I'd like.

Looking at him now, it's hard to believe he was only two and a half pounds at birth. He looked more like a frog than a human being. That was quite a time. I can conjure up that day by simply closing my eyes and invoking its memory. All the sensation of that bygone hour easily flows through me.

It was early fall. Summer's sunlight left an afterglow as the leaves turned yellow and orange. The air was brisk and clean with a pleasing aroma. Soon we would steady ourselves for winter's call. It was time to enjoy the wonder of nature turning the page. These marvelous moments that delight the senses and stir fond memories also illuminate the gateway toward tomorrow.

Not long after our fourth miscarriage, Carolyn and I found ourselves pregnant again. Determined and hopeful, our emotions soared. Just like the four previous times, we joyfully felt that this was it.

We decided to keep the news to ourselves for a while because we didn't want to raise the hopes of our families. While our parents and siblings anxiously awaited the arrival of the next generation, their hope had faded with each ensuing miscarriage. It would be hard to go through their disappointment and sympathy again. But Carolyn and I are not secretive, so within a month, our families were given the news that we hoped to have a child in the summer.

In spite of being classified a high-risk pregnancy, we could not contain our optimism. Early fall rolled into November, then December. Each week we visited Dr. Lewis. With each passing day, we dared believe that our dream would come true.

On January 3, 1984, we had an appointment to have a sonogram. It was a cold but sunny morning. All the leaves that littered the streets and driveways from autumn's fall had blown away. Like every prospective parent of our generation, we looked at a sonogram as a prenatal milestone. It was a milestone that we had never successfully reached before. Excited and nervous, Carolyn swelled her body with 20 ounces of water, a most uncomfortable prerequisite; and we made our way to the lab.

Sitting in the waiting room, my nervousness gave way to thirst. I went over to the water cooler for a drink, only to find an entire room filled with women who were looking at me in disbelief. I quickly took my seat, half feeling guilty and half hoping that what I perceived as my insensitivity was all in my mind.

The nurse called Carolyn in and my fear heightened considerably. Carolyn was uneasy too. She got up, kissed me on the cheek, and said with a nervous smile, "Wish us luck." I told her, "Don't worry. Everything's going to be just fine." I was left behind to wonder and imagine what she was about to go through.

While anxiously waiting, my mind began to drift. I floated in suspended time and happily recalled a winter's day when I was a child. My sister and I had just been outside playing in the snow as my father briskly shoveled the front walk. Debbie and I were soaking wet and chilled to the bone. My mom huddled us around the radiator with a cup of hot chocolate and wrapped us in wool flannel blankets. We watched wide-eyed out the front window as the snow continued to fly down from the sky. My dad came in right behind us. We all laughed at him because he had little icicles hanging from his mustache. After he took off his hat and coat and pulled off his boots, he joined us by the front window. My father put his arms around my mom and Debbie and I and hugged all of us. We cuddled together experiencing the warmth of family. It's that feeling that I now wished to feel as a husband and father.

"Mr. Liebling, you can come in now." Finally, I was called in. Apprehensively, I made my way down a long dimly lit hall, rhythmically praying with each step, that we could still dream the dream of family and not revisit the nightmare of pregnancies past.

As I walked into a dark room, I saw Carolyn lying down on a table looking at a monitor. The doctor stood next to her. When she heard me come into the room, she smiled and softly said, "Come over here and look at your baby's heartbeat."

With those words, a thousand thoughts blended into one. I was afraid to look at the monitor. I was afraid the heartbeat wouldn't be there. I was afraid that if I looked, the heartbeat would disappear.

Hesitantly, I walked over to the monitor and saw a pulse on the screen.

"There it is, Carolyn," I said. "Look at that!" We smiled at each other, held hands, and together we enjoyed that moment. We lingered there for as long as we could daring to dream about bringing a child into the world.

Filled with thanks to reach this point, we went home.

Dr. Lewis ordered Carolyn to stay in bed for the rest of the pregnancy. Weekly visits to his office were scheduled on the calendar. The baby was due July 23rd. As the next few months passed, there were an assortment of complications to navigate.

We watched as Carolyn's belly grew. Dr. Lewis allowed us to go through Lamaze classes. It was there that I noticed that Carolyn was carrying the baby smaller than the rest of the other pregnant women in the class.

June 9th was a warm sunny day. The sky was pale baby blue without a hint of a cloud. I took the morning off from work to take Carolyn for another sonogram. We both thought it routine. We found out later that Dr. Lewis was also concerned that Carolyn was carrying too small. So off we went to the doctor's office, thinking that everything was fine.

When we returned, I dropped Carolyn off at home and went back to work. Several hours later, about 1:00 P.M., Carolyn called me and said that she just got off the phone with Dr. Lewis.

"Is everything all right?" I asked.

She said that Dr. Lewis wanted us to go to the hospital to do what he called a non-stress test.

"What the heck is that?" I asked.

"Dr. Lewis is concerned that the baby is too small and there seems to be a smaller than usual amount of amniotic fluid."

So I hurriedly left work. I got into my car, which was parked in a municipal parking lot. I was headed for the exit when I got stuck behind another car. The driver had one foot out of the car and was arguing with the driver of another car who was trying to enter the parking lot. The two of them were yelling back and forth. Neither one of them wanted to give in and let the other pass.

Well, something came over me. I got out of my car and went over to the two drivers and yelled out, "My wife is having a baby. Stop arguing so I can get out of here." Without hesitation, they got back into their cars and parted like the Red Sea—and I was on my way.

As I headed for the parkway, I was musing at my parking lot escape. I decided that this was a good dress rehearsal for next month when the baby was due.

When I got home, Carolyn was waiting for me. We gathered ourselves and quickly went off–all the time wondering "What do you think is happening?" On the ride to the hospital, I told Carolyn what happened in the parking lot and we both laughed nervously.

When we reached the hospital, I drove around to the front, dropped Carolyn off, and went to park the car. When I returned, I was surprised to learn that Carolyn was being admitted into the hospital. She was answering all the usual administrative questions and they gave her an ID bracelet.

At that moment, it dawned on me that this was not a dress rehearsal after all. With the baby due a month and a half from now and our history of unhappy results, I started to become extremely concerned. We met Dr. Lewis in a small room on the maternity floor. He asked Carolyn to get undressed and slip on the traditional hospital gown. He left the room for a moment to give her privacy.

He returned with urgency in his eyes and immediately began to attach Carolyn to an assortment of machines. When he finished, he turned on the machines and announced that he'd be back in twenty minutes. Before he left, he briefed us.

"This test will tell us if the baby is in distress," he said.

"What if that happens?" I nervously asked.

"If the baby is under too much stress, it would be better for the baby's survival to be out of the womb."

"Does that mean you might deliver the baby sooner than later?" I asked.

"Yes, but we'll try to prolong it as long as possible," he said.

I had no response.

"Okay, then, I'll be back in twenty minutes," he said as he left the room.

I went over to Carolyn and began to look at all the machines that were attached to her. There were beeps and charts and graphs and I investigated each one of them as if I could tell what was happening. I could see that Carolyn was getting terribly nervous.

"Will I be all right? she asked. "What's going to happen to the baby?" she asked, not waiting for a response to her first question.

"Everything is going to be just fine, you'll see," I said. I was trying to comfort both of us.

"We're in good hands. Dr. Lewis is a fine doctor. He knows what he's doing," I said, hoping that would soothe us.

The next twenty minutes seemed to go by so slowly. But when Dr. Lewis came walking into the room, I wanted those twenty minutes back. My anxiety level rose. He went over to Carolyn and softly asked, "Is everything all right?" She nodded her head yes.

Dr. Lewis started to check all the graphs and charts. We all knew we arrived at an impending crossroad. We suffered the anticipation in silence. The air in the room felt like it was closing in on us. That moment practically took our breath away.

Dr. Lewis seemed to be hanging in suspended animation. Then, as if reconnected with real time, he announced, "We're going to have a baby today!"

"What? Now?"

"Yes, now," he said calmly. "The baby is in distress and will do better outside the womb than in. I'll be right back with Dr. Rivers. She'll tell you what's going to happen."

With that, he quickly left the room. I was stunned. Carolyn immediately asked me if everything was going to be all right. I said, "Of course! We're in good hands." But she was scared and so was I.

Within a few moments, a small, determined woman walked in the room. Dr. Lewis was right behind her. He stepped forward and introduced Dr. Rivers, a neonatal specialist.

"Dr. Rivers will explain some things to you," he said.

What was to follow assaulted us. It was a barrage of unhappy possibilities. Our baby, whom we had nurtured for six months in Carolyn's womb, was in real distress. There wasn't enough amniotic fluid. The baby could be born without kidneys. In addition, it could be hard for the baby to breathe on its own.

My composure started to break down. My emotions rose to the surface. As my heart sank, tears filled my eyes. My poor baby. My poor Carolyn. Why was this happening? Is what they're saying true?

A stream of illogical thoughts pierced my mind one after the other. Maybe the baby had a genetic disorder that Debbie might have had. I immediately thought that this was my fault. Suddenly I felt helpless. Irrationally I thought, I don't even have a kidney to donate.

Dr. Rivers' comments were filled with could be's and maybes. Do I dare think other than the worst? This is not the way it's supposed to be. None of this happened to anyone that I knew. The magnitude of an unknown consequence bore down on us.

Dr. Rivers said a few more things, but my ears were already ringing. She asked us if Carolyn had alcohol or smoked cigarettes during her pregnancy, both of which she had not. The damage to my sensibilities had already been done. I couldn't absorb another "thing." As quickly as she came, Dr. Rivers was gone. Dr. Lewis remained and indicated that it was time to prepare for an emergency Cesarean section. He left Carolyn and I alone to console each other.

Carolyn momentarily became brave and optimistic and I tried

to put up a good front too. But I was severely shaken. Carolyn told me to call her mom and I decided to also call my sister. My parents were out of the country on vacation. On the way to the telephone, I broke down and I couldn't contain the tears. When I called our families, they were shocked but supportive. On the way back to Carolyn, I knew I had to compose myself for her sake.

It was time. I told her not to worry and that everything was going to turn out fine. She and I had traveled a long distance together. The road had been bumpy but we were there for each other every step of the way. Now, here at the defining moment, we were being separated. The doctor wouldn't allow me to be in the operating room. As we walked this lap into the unknown, we comforted each other. I was scared for her, for the baby, and for myself.

Carolyn held my hand and asked, "Who's going to watch out for me?" Dr. Lewis stretched out his hand and said, "Hold onto my hand. I have good hands to hold." With that, I kissed my wife good-bye and said, "I'll see you soon. Be brave." She smiled at me with a tear in her eye and said, "I love you." Almost inaudibly and choking back a tear, I said, "I love you, too."

As I watched my wife being wheeled into the operating room, I felt alone—truly alone. What will happen to us if things don't work out? I began to pray to God harder than I ever had before. Tears filled my eyes as I paced back and forth. Please let everything be okay. Please let my baby be healthy. Please don't let anything bad happen to Carolyn. Please don't hurt us.

These moments will stay with me forever. Looking back, through all the emotions, somehow the message got through. Everything was going to be all right. With every step, I prayed harder. Deep down inside from the center of my being came a feeling that we were going to make it. I know that seems like a contradiction, but through my anxiety, and through the fear, there was a sense that someone or something was watching over us. I wasn't alone any more.

It seemed like I was waiting in the hallway forever when a nurse finally came out. I hope it's all over and everything's okay, I thought to myself.

"Are you Mr. Liebling?" she asked me.

"Yes, I am. Is everything okay?" I asked.

"Yes, everything is fine. We're about to begin."

"You haven't started yet?" I asked, half astonished and half frustrated.

"No, not yet, but it shouldn't take too long," she said with a reassuring smile.

"Okay, please have someone come out and let me know what's happening as soon as possible. I'll be waiting here," I said.

She went back to the operating room and I went back to pacing. Within a short while, I found myself racing down the hall with a nurse and a portable incubator.

"It's a boy!" she said.

"Oh, my God. Is he all right?"

"He scored a perfect APGAR, and he looks fine. We have to take him to the preemie nursery to have the doctors check him out from head to toe."

"How is my wife? She's okay, right?"

"She's just fine. She's concerned about you."

"When can I see her?"

"They're not done with the 'C' section. You can stay with the baby and we'll come and get you when she's in the recovery room."

We practically ran down the hall to the preemie nursery. That's where they keep all the premature babies. When we arrived, I was pretty startled to see a high-tech room where teams of doctors and nurses were running around from station to station. Babies were hooked up to all types of machines.

They brought my baby to one of those stations and within seconds, a swarm of doctors and nurses stood around him. I couldn't really see what was going on. They blocked my view. I looked on anxiously. Then, a woman in a mask and gown turned around and gave me the thumbs up sign. I realized that it was Dr. Rivers.

As she came to the door that I was peering through, she had a big smile on her face. My dread and worry melted away. I knew we had made it. My heart raced with joy. She opened the door and told me the words I longed for.

"Everything is going to be all right. He's going to be just fine. He's a little guy, only two and a half pounds. He's going to have to stay here for a few weeks until he grows."

"He can breathe on his own?

"Yes."

"His kidneys are okay?"

"He has already peed."

"Thank you, Dr. Rivers."

"Would you like to see him?"

"I can?"

"Yes, follow me. You'll have to put on this mask and gown."

The last time I put on a gown like that was to see my sister after the transplant.

I followed her to the end of the room where there was a rocking chair. She told me to sit down. I did and a nurse handed me my son wrapped in a diaper. He was so tiny and delicate that I was almost afraid he would roll off my hand if I breathed too hard. I looked at him and raised him closer to me. I whispered, "I love you." Then something funny occurred to me. He looked very familiar. I couldn't quite place it. Then it dawned on me; he looked just like me.

A knock came on the viewing glass behind me. It was my sister smiling from ear to ear. As I smiled back, I carefully tilted my baby up for Debbie to get a better look. Still smiling, she mouthed the words, "He looks just like me." I looked at her and then at him again and I saw she was right. The baby had a strong resemblance to the two of us. At that moment we shared in the gift of life and renewal. Intuitively, I felt a circle close. By donating my kidney to Debbie, she was able to be with me to share that moment. Because of my gift, she was alive to experience the miracle and gift of another life. Having her there connected the miracle of the past to the miracle of that day and pointed to the hope of tomorrow. I lowered the baby to my lap and looked down at my son again. As his chest rhythmically drew in the breath of life, my heart brimmed with gratitude.

I held onto that moment long and hard. Debbie knocked on the window again and waved goodbye because she had to go back to work. As she walked away, a nurse came over to tell me that Carolyn was in the recovery room and that I could see her. I told my son I would see him soon, and that I had to go visit with his mother.

I handed the baby back to the nurse, who took him and placed him in his station. I told Dr. Rivers that I was going to see my wife and I would see her later. I thanked her again. I was walking a good foot off the ground. I couldn't wait to see Carolyn.

A nurse walked me to the recovery room.

"Carolyn, Carolyn, how are you?"

"I'm doing fine," she said in a semi-drowsy state.

"I just came from the baby. He's wonderful. They say he's

going to be all right."

"I know. Dr. Lewis sent someone down to the nursery to find out. Do you think he'll be all right?" she asked.

"I held him in my arms. He's so tiny, but Dr. Rivers said he's strong. He'll have to stay in the preemie nursery to gain weight. He's only two and a half pounds. They say that the next 48 hours are critical, but I know he's going to be all right."

"Oh, Larry, he's so tiny. I don't think he'll make it. I'm so scared."

It was then that I realized that Carolyn's experience was quite different from mine. When they wheeled her into the operating room, she was scared and filled with fright. Dr. Lewis held her hand and tried to soothe her. While I was outside worrying about her and the baby about to be born, she was undergoing major surgery. While it was an assault on me mentally and emotionally, it was that and more for her. She was also physically threatened. That leaves you with quite a different perspective. She was scared that she or the baby or both of them would die.

"Tell me what happened to you," I said.

"They wheeled me into the operating room. Immediately, Dr. Lewis started to prepare for the surgery. There were so many monitors beeping. Larry, I was so nervous. I wished you were there. I felt that no one was watching out for me. I felt so alone. The funny thing, though, is that after a while, I felt that I was going to be all right. But I wasn't so sure about the baby. Are you sure he's all right?"

"Yes, he's wonderful. Didn't they show you him? How was he born?"

"Everything happened very quickly. They told me they were about to start. Before I knew it, I heard a baby crying. Dr. Lewis told me it was a boy. He then said, 'He looks good, he looks good!' Tears rolled down my cheeks. Could you believe it? I was still wearing my glasses. They kept steaming up. Then a nurse brought the baby next to me. All I could think about was whether he was going to live. Dr. Lewis came over to me and asked if I was all right. I said yes. He gave me a kiss and congratulated me. I told Dr. Lewis that his name would be Joshua. Then a nurse scooped up the baby and rolled him out of the room."

"You've been through a lot, sweetie," I said, trying to ease her apprehension. I could see that she was still very concerned about the baby's condition. Maybe I was naive, but I felt that everything was all right now.

"Everything happened so quickly. I can't believe it. When we came here this afternoon, I thought it would be a good dress rehearsal," I said.

"That seems so long ago. It's hard to believe this all happened in one day."

Just then, Dr. Lewis came into the room. I thanked him over and over again. Carolyn asked, "How is the baby?" The doctor said that he's doing very well. He told us that he'll look in on the baby from time to time, but Dr. Rivers was the expert when it came to the baby's condition. He told Carolyn that her room was ready for her and it would be a good idea for her to get some rest. Then he looked at us and said, "You two really love each other." Carolyn and I smiled at each other. I kissed her on the head and told Dr. Lewis, "Thank you. Thank you for everything you've done. Without you, I don't know what would have happened."

It's wonderful how in some moments we can transcend the din of the ordinary. The three of us somehow shared the power of that moment and found it sublime. While that day's impact will affect Carolyn and I for the rest of our lives, Dr. Lewis was also moved by the part he played. The three of us had been through something together and recognized the miracle and mystery of it all.

Dr. Lewis bid us goodnight. The attendant came to take Carolyn to her room. I walked alongside her down the hall basking in the aftermath of the day's events. Everything seemed illuminated. Carolyn quietly got settled. We were careful not to wake the woman in the next bed. It was 12:30 A.M.

Carolyn started to drift off to sleep, so I said good-night. It was time to go home. Tomorrow would hold the promise of a whole new life together. I walked out of the hospital exhausted, but exhilarated at the same time. In the sky, the stars shimmered. A warm breeze gently caressed me. I looked up into the night, raised my arms, and said, "Thank you, God. Thank you for being there with us."

While the next month held some trying moments that were not expected, our son came home with us on July17th. My life would not be the same without Joshua. For Carolyn and I, he almost wasn't. The fact that life is a mystery is no surprise. The surprise, though, is sometimes we say it and don't really feel it. The miracle of Joshua's birth leaves me forever grateful and in awe of birth and growth.

Children are the greatest gift God can bestow on us. He gives us these little beings to nourish and in return we are nourished ourselves. He asks us to teach them how to experience their lives and fulfill their promise and in return, we are fulfilled.

It wasn't long ago that my little Josh fell asleep watching TV in the family room. Maybe he was ten at the time. It had been awhile since the last time I remember him doing that. So when I picked him up to carry him off to his bed, I was quite surprised to discover that my little boy was bigger and heavier than I remembered. Once so light and easy to papoose anywhere, now he was

145

more arms and legs than I could recall.

As I slowly put him down on his bed, I felt a rush of emotions spring up from the center of my soul. I was both happy and sad. Happy that my boy was growing up so strong in his mind, body, and spirit. But I was sad, too, for myself, because in that instant, I realized it would not be long before he was completely grown and gone from our nest. It would not be long before the cocoon of three souls in safe harbor would give way to a different reality.

The truth is that life is always changing. We are forever bound to the cycles of birth, death, and renewal that allow us to experience our own being. I think we are always on the move. Sometimes we doom ourselves to repeat the same lesson in different ways. In some fundamental way, deep down, we set ourselves up that way. It's like a self-imposed drama that we star in until we eventually break through to some revealed truth. Then life unfolds anew and so it goes. Layer after layer is peeled away and life's fruit is laid bare for us to taste and savor. So it is for us and so it is for our children.

"This is Carolyn. We're not in right now but if you leave your name and number, we'll get back to you."

I was completely unaware that the phone rang.

"Larry, are you there? It's me." It was Carolyn. "I'm in the car and I'll pick up Josh on the way home." She was leaving a message from the car phone.

I ran inside to pick up the phone.

"Carolyn!" I said.

"Oh, you're home. I thought maybe you took Molly for a walk after all."

"No, I just couldn't get to the phone in time," I said.

"I'll pick up Joshua on my way home," she repeated.

"Maybe you should call to see if he's ready to leave Matt's house?" I suggested.

"He's been out for awhile, and I think it's time to come home," she said.

"It seems like he just left. What time is it?" I asked.

"It's four o'clock already," she answered.

"I didn't realize that time was moving so fast. I still think you should call first."

"Better yet, I have a couple of more stops I can make. That will give Josh plenty of time and I can get a few extra things done.

"Sounds good to me. I'll see you in a bit," I said and went back outside.

Part Three:
Late Afternoon
Same Day
September 1, 1996

❖ ❖ ❖ ❖

15

❖ ❖ ❖ ❖

As the afternoon sun softened, the day's heat noticeably dissolved into a cool breeze. I briefly thought about going inside, but within a short while, my body adjusted comfortably to the new temperature. It's hard to believe that I've been sitting here since morning. Molly jaunts over to me to say hello and to be sure that I didn't forget that she was still with me.

"Hello, girl, you're such a good dog. You kept me company all day. I guess we should have gone for a walk. We could have both used the exercise." She looked at me with her ears perking up as I said the word "walk," as if I made some kind of contractual agreement to stroll around the neighborhood at the mere mention of the word.

"Maybe later we'll go, girl. Right now, let's just hang out here."

Molly just turned four this past May. From the start, she was the sweetest dog and family friend. Today was no different. She stayed by my side as I culled through my feelings. My heart felt full as I thought about Joshua and Carolyn. My life has been full of grace. Looking back at it now, it seems as if someone had always been looking after me. There have been many moments when things have looked bleak, but have turned out for the best.

Yet, like a dark dour cloud that shrouds the brilliance of the midday sky, life rarely goes in one direction. A patch of darkness too often can blot out the sun's glory. So, too, my full heart bares sorrow with the hope that healing comes sooner than later.

As easily as the wind changes direction, so did my backyard mood shift decidedly somber. I began to think about the last year and the trials that my sister endured.

Debbie was a very important part of our family life. She was a wonderful aunt to Joshua and would marvel at each of Joshua's milestones. She saw in Joshua an opportunity to be a mentor and wanted to be an integral part of his life. A week wouldn't go by without her visiting. Friday night dinners always meant running around the house playing ball or hide and seek–Molly getting into the act as well.

Debbie and Carolyn had become close friends and talked all the time. They would talk for hours discussing anything from what happened at work to exchanging recipes for pecan pie.

Contrary to our teenage years, Debbie and I would often exchange music and laugh about something either my mother or father did or said that was funny. We went to baseball games, movies, and restaurants. We shared investment strategies and I helped her weigh different ideas about starting her own business.

Debbie lived alone for eleven years in a house that she rented in Babylon. I could never quite understand how she was able to do that for so long. It always seemed so lonely to me. I think it got to her at times, but she never expressed it to me. Carolyn often told me that she thought that a part of Debbie enjoyed living alone and that I was placing my lifestyle choices on her. But I was always left with the feeling she wanted more.

I always thought that Debbie had another side to her that was neatly tucked away from the family but available to her friends. Perhaps that's the way it is for a lot of people–not feeling free enough to show their multifaceted selves to their immediate family. Perhaps it becomes easier to assume the role expected of us. At times I would wonder what were the other sides of my sister.

She didn't have any trouble with the transplant. For twenty-one years, she took her medication and the thought of rejection, although not too far below the surface, faded into the background.

It seemed as if Debbie was finally getting her life together. She was the happiest I had seen her in a long time. She had saved enough money to put a down payment on a house and was already beginning the search to buy her own home.

Her professional career was on the move, too. She converted a room in the house she rented in Babylon into an office and opened a part-time psychologist practice. She was also extremely excited about a new idea she had formulated. She identified a niche in the health care industry that required an accomplished personnel advisor and placement counselor. She felt confident that she could fulfil that role and was on the verge of establishing her own corporation to see it to fruition.

The only fly in the ointment was physical. She began to complain about lower back problems. At first, she was given pain-killers and muscle relaxants. They helped somewhat but she continued to be plagued with discomfort. She spent over a year going to several doctors to see if anyone could help. One doctor found large fibrous growths in her uterus and thought that maybe it was putting pressure on her back. With all the proper precautions and a kidney transplant specialist on hand, Debbie had a hysterectomy. The operation was successful but it wasn't a cure. She had three months of relief and then began to complain of more back pain.

One early autumn day, I met Debbie and my parents for lunch. When I arrived at the diner, my parents and sister were already there. Carolyn had a business meeting and couldn't join us. My father already was sipping a cup of coffee. For my dad, what made a restaurant worthy of a second visit was a good cup of coffee and food that was served hot and fast.

"Hi Mom, Hi Dad, Hi Deb," I said as I walked up to the table.

"Hi dear. Your sister and I just got here. Your father came straight from the office." My mom kissed me hello.

We all perused the menu even though we knew it by heart. The waiter came over and we all ordered. After he left, we began to catch up with what was going on in our lives. My mom and dad had just come back from a vacation in New Mexico and were reviewing all the sights and sounds of their southwestern sojourn. I updated everyone on how Josh was making out with the new school year.

Then someone yelled over from another table, "Hey, Debbie, how you doing?" She winced in pain as she twisted to see who it was, her back obviously still hurting her.

"Who's that?" I asked.

"Someone I know from work," she said.

"What's wrong with you?" my mom asked with concern.

"Mom, you know my back is still hurting me."

"I thought the surgery was supposed to correct that," my father said, simultaneously picking up his cup of coffee for another sip.

"I thought so too, but it's back."

"Didn't you go to another doctor a couple of weeks ago?" I asked.

"Yes. He said I probably pulled a muscle. He doesn't think the pain is from the same source as before. I'm not so sure he's right, though, because the pain is pretty much in the same spot as before the hysterectomy. He gave me some painkiller and some muscle relaxant, but I still feel the pain and, in fact, I think it's getting worse. I'm getting a little frustrated over the whole thing. No one seems to be able to tell me what it is."

"Why don't you see another doctor, then?" my mom interjected.

"I already have an appointment to see someone else."

"When is it? I could go with you if you want."

"No thanks, Mom. My appointment is tomorrow and I can go by myself."

Debbie had become accustomed to my mother's constant concern. Sometimes, I think she wanted it, looked for it, and needed it desperately. Yet at other times, she felt annoyed at my mom's involvement and what she perceived as her own dependence. Debbie and my mother had a unique and complicated relationship, which was woven together by many life-worn emotional threads. It is hard to determine what their relationship would have been had Debbie not gotten sick at such a young age. Nothing happens in a vacuum. It is tinged with the drama that develops between people. My mother nurtured her through the most trying moments life can tender. Debbie accepted, needed, and wanted that attention. Often behavior becomes habitual as a pattern is set and programmed in. Then it can run all the time regardless of circumstance. I don't think Debbie or my mother could change the nature of their relationship even as my sister reached the ages of twenty, thirty, thirty-five, or even as she reached age forty.

When you arrive at a certain age, everyone seems to develop back problems. I guess the accumulated stress of our rushed lives leave a lot of us searching for relief from physical pain. In my family, it was no different. My mother, father, Carolyn, and I all at one time or another pulled muscles or slipped discs. So we were all very familiar with back pain. Now as my sister reached the advanced age of 39, I guess we all thought that it was her turn. She probably just had to give it some time and it would go away.

The rest of lunch was the usual fare. My father and I talked about how bad the Giants had become again. My mother bothered my sister by probing to see if she had any "dates" lately. As is their custom, my mother and father argued about where they were going for dinner. My mother stopped cooking dinner on a regular basis a few years earlier. It wasn't that they really argued; they just couldn't make up their mind where to go, so they got on each other's nerves.

"Where do you want to go, Eddie? It's up to you, because I don't really care." This was always my mom's opening line.

"Well, I don't really care either, so you make up your mind." My father would always toss the ball back into my mother's court.

"Eddie, please stop it already and decide where you want to go. I know you really do care where we go and I don't. So you decide." They would volley a few rounds.

It went on like that for a few minutes more before I suggested that they go to Dominic's for Italian food. They both thought that was a great idea.

Debbie said she had to leave. She gave us all a kiss and said that she'd speak to us tomorrow after her doctor's appointment. We all wished her luck.

16

❖ ❖ ❖ ❖

"Debbie, is that you? Calm down. I can't hear what you're saying," Carolyn said, trying to soothe Debbie's agitated state.

My sister was still having terrible trouble with her back. Her doctors had sent her for every test you could imagine. She had resisted taking an MRI because she wasn't sure how it would affect the kidney. Since she had taken every other kind of test and received inconclusive results, she decided to do the MRI.

Now, she was calling with the results.

"Larry, get on the extension. Your sister is on the phone and she's very upset," Carolyn yelled to me from the kitchen.

I quickly rushed to the phone. Debbie was calling from her home.

"Hi, Deb. How are you doing?"

"Not so good. The doctor just called with the MRI results."

"What's the matter?"

"He said there's some kind of growth on my sacrum."

"What kind of growth?"

"It may be cancer."

"Where's the sacrum?"

"At the base of the spine."

I was stunned by what she said. Never in my wildest dreams did I think that her problems would stem from something like that. I thought maybe a ruptured disc, a muscle pull, but cancer, never.

"Could it be some other kind of growth? Something benign?"

"He said it could be. He wasn't sure. He said the only way to find out for sure is to have a biopsy."

"Is he going to do that?"

"No. He's sending me to a specialist in Baltimore."

"When?"

"As soon as I can make arrangements."

"Larry, will you please call the doctor to make sure I heard everything right? This whole thing is impossible to believe. I felt my heart in my throat when he said cancer. I told him you might call."

"Absolutely! I'll call him right now. What's his name?"

"Dr. Nicholas."

"Okay, give me his number."

"555-9409."

"Call him now. He should be there. I just spoke to him."

With that, Debbie hung up. I was trying to gather my thoughts before I called. Carolyn and I looked at each other in disbelief. I started to write down some of the questions that were rolling around in my head. Then I decided to just call. Debbie was right; the doctor was in and expecting my call.

"Dr. Nicholas, my sister asked me to call you. I understand that she had an MRI and it shows that she has some sort of growth."

"I'm afraid, she may have a cancerous chordoma. A lot of the time, this type of cancer is found in people who have taken certain immuno-suppressant drugs. More often than not, it's found on the base of the brain and then there's nothing we can do. In your sister's case, it's at the base of her spine on the sacrum and I'm hoping something can be done. I'm sending her to someone who I feel is the right doctor in this type of situation. He'll do a biopsy and we'll know more."

"Could it be a benign tumor?"

"Yes, that's possible, but I'd be less than honest with you if I told you that was the way I'm expecting this thing to go."

"Is my sister going to die?"

"There is always that possibility." He dazed me with his direct response.

"But perhaps with surgery, she'll be all right?" I quickly interjected.

"Yes, of course. We really have to do a biopsy to see what we are dealing with."

"Okay, Dr. Nicholas. Thanks for your time. Can I call you if I have any further questions?"

"Anytime."

My eyes started to tear as I thought of the possibility of losing my sister. But I was determined not to let my emotions run rampant. There was a task at hand and I felt the best way to handle everything was one day at a time. So I called my sister back to report that she had indeed heard him right. She was in for a fight and no one knew what the result would be. Debbie had fought and won before. Twenty-two years had passed since the onset of her last major battle–a victory she celebrated with life renewed every day. Call it wishful thinking, but I was hopeful that she would be the victor here, too.

Then I became very anxious. How was I going to tell my parents?

17

❖ ❖ ❖ ❖

It turned out that I didn't have to tell my folks. They knew that Debbie was scheduled to get the MRI results so my mother called her first.

My mom worried about Debbie every day since the transplant. There wasn't a day that went by that my mom didn't ask me if I heard from her. How was she? Was she feeling okay? Was anything troubling her? She would ask Carolyn the same regimen of questions. She was looking for the slightest clue as to the quality of Debbie's life. Most of the time, there was nothing to worry about. Now, unfortunately, there was.

We all became mobilized. My parents made arrangements to go to Baltimore with Debbie for her biopsy. It was expected that the biopsy would keep Debbie in the hospital overnight, two days at the most.

Debbie immediately went to a health food store and bought vitamins and macrobiotic food, along with a juicer and recipe books for cooking a vegetarian diet.

Carolyn started to call around her extensive network of

friends, relatives, and neighbors for advice and to see if anyone had a similar experience. I tried to keep calm and urged everyone to take one day at a time. I felt it was my job to try to keep the situation from getting out of control. I guess a part of me was afraid to see my sister and parents hurting from the emotional trauma. Even though things were serious, we weren't one hundred percent sure that it was cancer. There was always a chance that Dr. Nicholas could be wrong.

Debbie was pretty frightened, but she also was determined to get to the bottom of what was wrong with her and to get the proper treatment so that she could go on with her life. We all talked about our fears but we tried to be optimistic at the same time.

They were leaving Monday for the hospital and we planned to go out for dinner the night before. It was kind of a tradition in my family that anytime something major happened, we'd go out to dinner. Whether it was a birthday, anniversary, holiday, or one of us going on vacation, we'd go out together, and it always revolved around a meal.

As we asked the waiter for the check, we began the usual countdown to saying good-bye.

"Dad, don't worry about the business. I'll look in on it while you're away."

"Okay, I appreciate that," he said.

"Never mind the business! Be sure to take care of my dog and cat," Debbie said. Carolyn and I agreed to look after Debbie's dog, Samantha, and her cat, Chelsea.

"Don't worry, Aunt Deb. I'll remind them," Josh said.

"And who's going to remind you?" Carolyn said to Josh.

"Very funny, Mom. You know I have a better memory than you do."

"Yeah? Is that why I have to remind you to do your home-work, brush your teeth, go to sleep, go to the...?"

"Mom, that's enough! Besides, you don't have to make such a big deal out of it."

"That's enough, you two. It's time for everybody to say good-bye," I said.

As we kissed and hugged and said our good-byes, a rush of emotions swelled through all of us. It was as if the landscape of our lives was changing right before our eyes.

We walked out to our respective cars. Watching them pull out of the parking lot, I could feel my heartstrings ache. I felt sep-arated from them, but quickly figured that they would be home in a couple of days. Hopefully, they would get better than expected results.

As I started the car, raindrops began to dot the front window. The wind kicked up and the night crashed with the sound of distant thunder. Then a flash brightened the sky and the rain be-gan to beat rhythmically on the roof of the car. The windshield wipers soon sang a hypnotic tune as the rain streamed down the windows. As we drove away silently in the pouring rain, I began to pray:

"God, watch over them. Please don't let anything bad hap-pen. Let Debbie not have cancer. Let it be some sort of growth that can be taken care of easily without too much pain." Wiping a tear from my face, I prayed, "God, don't let Debbie die."

18

❖ ❖ ❖ ❖

"Dad, how's Debbie? Did everything go all right?"

"They finished the biopsy and your sister is in recovery."

"When will they have the results?"

"They won't know for at least three or four days. They will probably know on Thursday."

"When do you think you'll be coming home?"

"She'll have to stay here for a day or two."

"How are you and Mom?"

"We're both nervous about the results. I don't think we'll get any relief until we know what we're dealing with. Of course once we know, that will start a whole different cycle of worry. What a thing to happen to her! Didn't she go through enough with the kidney thing?"

"Yeah, I know, but let's wait and see what's what. Maybe it won't be as bad as we think."

"I hope so but you know me, I always expect the worst."

"I know, but let's wait and see anyway. Does Mom want to say hello?"

"She's not here right now. She went to see if she could stay with Debbie in the recovery room."

"All right, Dad. Everything else is okay here. There are no major problems."

"Okay, I'll have your mother call you later."

"Fine. If there's any change, let us know."

"All right, Larry. I'll speak to you later. This is a hell of a thing to have happened."

"I'll talk to you later, Dad."

"What did he say?" Carolyn immediately asked when I hung up.

"They won't have any results for at least three or four days. They should be coming back in a couple of days."

"What else did he say? How's your mom? Did they see Debbie? Did they see the doctor? When will..."

"Hold on Ca, you're asking me too many questions."

"Sorry. You never get the whole story."

"My parents are fine, nervous, but they'll be all right."

"How come you didn't speak to your Mom?"

"She was trying to stay with Debbie. We'll know more to-morrow."

She was right, of course. Somehow she always gets more details than I do. I get the essentials and that's it. I don't know why that is, but it is. I think it's a male thing. Women are so used to talking on the telephone and finding out what's going on that when it comes to the details, they get it in color. Men tend to get the information and instantly internalize it; and you need a can opener to pry it out of us.

The next two days went by terribly slowly. I heard from my parents several more times. I spoke to Debbie and she was in a lot of pain. She wasn't able to go home because she couldn't get out of bed yet.

"I'm sure about it. I know it. I have cancer. I'm going to die," Debbie said over the phone.

"Come on Debbie. We don't know anything yet. You don't even have the results." I was trying to make her feel better.

"I know what I know," she said, having nothing to do with my positive outlook.

"Even if you have it, the doctors have told you they think they can remove it surgically."

"You don't understand. This is not a good situation." She was determined to have me agree.

"You're just nervous." I couldn't give into her.

"I'm also in a lot of pain. The woman next to me hasn't stopped crying since I came into this room."

"What's happened to her?" I asked.

"She had back surgery. How am I going to go through this?" she cried into the phone.

"Let's just take it one step at a time." It was getting hard to hold on to my wait-and-see attitude.

"How's Carolyn and Joshua?" she asked through her tears.

"Carolyn's right here. Do you want to speak to her?" I asked.

"Sure," she said.

Carolyn took the receiver from me and began to talk to Debbie. The truth is that I didn't know how she was going to get through this. She sounded miserable. I didn't know how my parents were going to get through this either. They were both getting older and I was worried about the strain on them.

We still didn't have the results. Nothing had really changed. The time waiting for the results of the biopsy was full of fear. I was very anxious for them to get back. Somehow, I wanted to believe that everything would be all right if only they could get out of the hospital, come home, and we'd sort the whole thing out.

Carolyn hung up with Debbie and looked at me with concern.

"What's going to happen to her? Your parents must be beside themselves."

"Let's just take one step at a time," I said. Her barrage of questions spun around in my head and all I wanted was a moment to clear my mind.

"Dr. Nicholas was wrong. It isn't a cancerous chordoma," my mother started off.

"It's not? What is it?" For a second, I let my spirits rise.

"It's worse. It's a neuro fibrosarcoma. It's an aggressive cancer," she said.

"Can they operate?" I asked.

"They can operate but there are complications."

"What sort of complications?"

"Oh, Larry! This is such a hard situation."

"What sort of complications, Mom?"

"She could lose some feeling in her feet and she may have to relearn how to go to the bathroom."

I couldn't respond.

"I was always so afraid that her kidney would reject. I never expected anything like this!" With that, my mother grimly said goodnight and hung up.

19

❖ ❖ ❖ ❖

On Thursday, Debbie and my parents came home from Baltimore. They had stayed longer than expected because Debbie was in too much pain to come home sooner. When they came back, they were all tired and apprehensive. The doctor who did the biopsy would also do the surgery. They all seemed to be pretty impressed with his credentials. It seems that he was one of the top orthopedic surgeons in the country. They also agreed that he didn't have much of a bedside manner.

"He's not becoming my best friend, but as long as he does the job, that's all I care about," my father confided in me.

They decided to do the operation and hope that none of the possible complications would come to pass. Everything was happening so fast; her surgery was immediately scheduled for the following Monday in Baltimore. Debbie was in a lot of pain and was determined to do what had to be done and get on with her life.

This was not going to be an easy surgery. A multitude of nerves run through the sacrum which made this an extremely delicate and risky venture. We had to be hopeful that the growth wasn't too large. The smaller the tumor, the less nerve damage there would be. The doctor would remove the growth and we'd all pray for the best. Though his promises were vague, the surgeon was confident he could minimize the possible damage.

The other question not yet fully addressed was whether the cancer had spread beyond the sacrum. All the tests Debbie had taken indicated that it had not, but we did not know for sure. We asked if she wanted to go for a second opinion, but she felt that she was being treated by one of the best and most capable doctors in the country.

It was a very long weekend. We all made arrangements to go down to Baltimore with Debbie for the surgery. My parents and Debbie would take the hour flight, and Carolyn and I decided to drive. We planned to leave Joshua home with friends overnight and be back the next day so that Josh wouldn't be without us for too long. He knew that his aunt was going into the hospital for difficult surgery and was very concerned. We wanted to be there for Debbie and my parents the day of the surgery but we felt that we couldn't stay long because we wanted to be sure that we were home for Josh, too.

Sunday arrived too quickly. Everyone was on edge, yet we all were trying to be as optimistic as possible. I remembered how well things went for Debbie with the transplant, and I hoped and envisioned a favorable result with this surgery as well.

Debbie and my parents were off to the airport. We dropped Josh off at school the usual time. Carolyn and I had a few things we had to take care of and then we would start out in the car.

During the car ride, we talked about Debbie. Somehow, I think we both felt that if we talked about it enough, everything would turn out all right. By the time Carolyn and I arrived, it was already dark. As it turned out, we arrived in Baltimore just about the same time as my parents and Debbie. Their plane was delayed and the usual quick trip turned out to be quite frustrating. Debbie was in pain and the added delay only aggravated her anxiety.

We all stayed at the Sheraton not far from Camden Yards where the Baltimore Orioles play baseball. You could see the stadium from our window and I thought it would have been nice to take a ride over if Josh was with us.

Carolyn and I were hungry so we went to a bar and grill located in the hotel. My father decided to join us. Debbie and my mom stayed in their room watching TV as they tried to relax.

My father was very concerned about the surgery. He had survived prostate cancer surgery four years earlier and was still aching from that experience. Cancer had become an all-encompassing and overriding worry for him. Carolyn and I tried to allay his fears; however, it's hard to be convincing when the same fears occupy your thoughts.

After we half-heartedly ate our dinner, we went back to the room where my mom and sister were resting. There we sat watching television. My sister played with a deck of cards. We noticed the hours pass, not saying much of anything. Frankly, I was uncomfortable. I wanted to be able to say something that would make everyone feel better but there were no words that could do that. Whatever I thought of had an empty ring to it in my mind.

Occasionally, someone would ask Debbie how she was feeling. She was still in quite a bit of pain from the biopsy and was taking medication to help her cope with the discomfort. The evening abruptly came to an end when my sister decided she wanted to try to get some sleep. Surgery was scheduled for first thing in the morning. It was hard to say goodnight. I gave her a kiss on the cheek. Silently I prayed, "God be with you."

171

Carolyn and I quietly went off to our room. The nighttime can be a comfort or a disquieting witness to the worried heart. I tossed and turned searching the night for a way out, for answers to questions that only echoed back in riddles. No one slept well that night and morning arrived with uneasiness. We gathered ourselves and met my parents and Debbie in the lobby of the hotel. The pre-dawn taxi ride through the streets of Baltimore was surreal. The early morning darkness cloaked any hint of the sunrise to follow. The wind wailed through a cracked window in the back seat.

I looked over at my sister and cried to myself. Why did she have to go through this? My mother and father looked anxious. Silently I tried to fight through a wall of worry with little success. We arrived at the hospital, checked in, and were ushered upstairs. Someone escorted us to a waiting area, where we were informed that the doctor wanted to speak with Debbie before the surgery.

Dr. Pratt was a tall man and walked in commanding an entourage, which followed obediently behind him. We all stood up as if a grand potentate had entered. My parents and Debbie greeted him and introduced him to Carolyn and myself. All of us sat down, and he took a seat next to Debbie. He cocked his head high, like a patrician peacock as he shuffled through a small stack of papers an assistant handed him. Looking over his reading spectacles which balanced perfectly on his long thin nose, it seemed as if he was looking down at us.

He said a few words to all of us. I asked a couple of questions about the surgery. How long will it be? He said between five and six hours. How long would Debbie be in the hospital? He indicated about two weeks. What kind of aftercare would she need? She might need some physical therapy. He then proceeded to whisper a few things to Debbie. As he did, I formed my opinion. I didn't like this man. I didn't trust him, and I felt uneasy about him. It didn't matter, though, because my sister had faith that this was the doctor that was going to save her from her cancer.

He left to prepare for surgery with his convoy of residents, secretaries, and nurses scrambling behind him. We asked Debbie what he had whispered to her. She shook her head as if to indicate that it wasn't important, just that he would make the necessary arrangements for therapy after the surgery to help her regain her mobility. Somehow I felt troubled. I didn't like the whispering. What was there to hide? I tried to ease my concerns. I surmised that maybe I was just being fearful for my sister and indeed I was. Yet something intuitively didn't feel right.

Debbie, though afraid, put on a brave face as she steadied herself to face the surgeon's knife. God, I prayed, guide the doctor's hand, and assist him in healing my sister. Let the cancer be contained and the damage be limited. Send us a miracle, protect her on her journey to the netherworld of infirmity, and return her to us unharmed.

It was time to get prepped for the operation. We were allowed to follow her to an area where they started to take blood pressure and temperature readings. Then they hooked her up to monitors. We all converged by Debbie's bedside. My mother held her hand in a scene that had an all too familiar air about it. We talked about all going on a Caribbean cruise together after Debbie recovered.

There we stood, half-reassuring Debbie, half-reassuring ourselves. If we could have willed her freedom from the bonds of her illness, it would be done. But if heaven had other plans, we'd be doomed to failure in the attempt.

The nurse came in and proclaimed the hour had arrived. We said our tearful good-byes and Debbie admonished us–not good-bye, just good luck.

We left her to travel on, alone. As we did, we were about to embark on a long day's voyage on a sea of uncertainty. We headed for the cafeteria for some coffee. The four of us talked about our hope for Debbie and tried to maintain an image of a bright tomorrow.

After the cafeteria, we went back upstairs to the waiting area with our books and magazines and newspapers. We all cast our eyes into the words we hoped would distract us long enough for the hours to pass by unnoticed. Several hours went by. Speaking softly, one of us would occasionally start a conversation about a relative or make an innocuous comment, trying to diffuse the tension. A random smile from someone else, waiting for a loved one, required a smile in kind.

Carolyn and I went to find a telephone to call our friends who were taking care of Joshua. He was fine and spent the night doing homework and then watching TV. We rejoined my parents in the waiting room. Shortly after, a doctor came in to talk to us. He specialized in kidneys. He told us that they had successfully isolated the kidney so that the operation could continue. Apparently, the kidney had to be moved aside so that the doctors could gain access to the sacrum.

When the doctor left, we looked at each other quizzically. None of us were informed that this was a concern. My father asked, "What else didn't they tell us?" We all agreed, though, at least they did what they had to and the procedure could continue.

Later in the afternoon, word came from the operating room that everything was going well; and the doctors were going to take a break. They suggested that we take a break as well and go down to the cafeteria for something to eat. We all looked at each other rather astonished. We had never heard of a medical team taking a break. We were hoping for the sign that it was over. Obviously, we had only reached some sort of medical halftime. But, at least everything was all right.

The four of us went downstairs to the cafeteria and ate a little something. Mostly, we needed a chance to stretch our legs. Carolyn also called home once again to let our friends know what was happening and to hear again that Joshua had a good night. When we returned to the waiting room an hour later, we were told that the surgery would resume shortly. All I could think of was let it be over already.

Hour after hour went by. Doctor after doctor came in to talk to other loved ones waiting. With each passing moment, we became more anxious. Day was turning to dusk. Our morning and afternoon waiting room companions had all left with their results. New faces entered the waiting room, as hours ticked away like days.

Carolyn struck up a conversation with a woman whose husband was also having surgery. They had come all the way from Wisconsin for a particular doctor. Her husband had a terrible problem with his back. There was only one doctor who could help him. She said this was the best hospital. People came from all over the world for the doctors here. That certainly sounded reassuring to us as we all listened in. What was the doctor's name? Dr. Pratt. We all said that couldn't be; there must be some mistake. We were stunned! The woman from Wisconsin was concerned for the fate of her husband, and the four of us all were wondering what was going on. I turned to Carolyn and said, "His assistants are doing part of someone's surgery. He can't be in two places at one time." She turned to me and said, "Yeah, but who's getting the short end of the stick?" I felt that he had betrayed a trust. My mom had asked him specifically before the surgery if he was doing the entire surgery and he answered yes.

Another hour passed. It was 8:00 P.M. Debbie was beginning her tenth hour of surgery. It was already twice as long as they told us it would be. Finally, Dr. Pratt came in looking worn and exhausted. He came over to us and immediately explained that he thought he had cut away all the cancer. The problem was that there was considerable nerve damage. He had cut nerves that controlled bladder and bowel function. He also cut away a nerve that controlled the upward movement of her left foot.

We were relieved to hear that Debbie was all right and had survived the surgery. When he said he had removed all the cancer, we also felt some solace. But when he told us that Debbie would have to learn how to control her bowel and bladder by means that weren't altogether clear to us, our hearts sank. Then he also told us she might need some additional surgery in the future to have bone grafts to build up her sacrum.

We all were very dazed and stunned. We were relieved to know that she had survived and hopefully was cancer free. But the problems that she was left with were beginning to add up to a considerable weight. What did it all mean?

Dr. Pratt presented all the consequences of the surgery in a calm manner. It was as if results were not insurmountable and within a short time, Debbie would be able to go back to her life. My father's eyes met mine. They seared with a mixture of emotions. His heart was torn apart from Debbie's suffering, but there was also anger at the cavalier way that the doctor discounted the difficulties. This was not going to be as easy as Dr. Pratt was making out. Debbie was traveling down a rough road and that meant we were all in for a hard time. We didn't say anything, but I knew we all felt it.

It further disturbed all of us when he said that Debbie might need additional surgery to build up her sacrum. What the hell did that mean? Did he know this beforehand?

While an impulse of distrust filtered through my mind, I wanted to be as optimistic for myself and for my parents as possible. I was very happy to know that she had survived the surgery, and the doctor felt he removed all of the cancer. I subdued any feeling of foreboding and willed my thoughts positive. I also decided that it was important to take one step at a time. Otherwise, everything would run away with itself, and I wanted to be a positive force during this whole thing.

My mother wanted to see Debbie before we went back to the hotel and asked the doctor if she could. He said that it would be better to come back in the morning. My mother thanked the doctor and off he went to talk to the woman from Wisconsin. I still didn't like or trust him.

Before the doctor left the waiting room, the woman from Wisconsin did ask him how he managed to do two surgeries at one time. He said that while one of his assistants did the closing surgery on Debbie, he was able to do her husband's operation. She was all smiles and must have received good news. I never quite bought his explanation.

20

❖ ❖ ❖ ❖

The next morning, after another restless night, we all got up early. Carolyn called the Intensive Care Unit at the hospital to find out how Debbie was doing. The nurse watching over her said she had moved her feet, and she felt it was a good sign that the nerves running to her feet were going to be all right.

We got dressed and met my parents in the lobby as we had the day before and off we went to the hospital to see my sister. The taxi ride over was one of relief that the surgery was over, but we were considerably apprehensive of what the immediate future held.

We walked into the hospital and found the Intensive Care Unit without a problem. The nurse charged with my sister's care led us to Debbie's bed. My heart wailed as I saw my sister seemingly grasping onto life. Tubes and electronic devices were everywhere. We circled her bed. Barely conscious, I am not even sure she knew we were there. Tearfully, one by one, we told her we loved her and that she was going to be all right. It was hard to control our emotions. It was as if she wasn't really there; only her ravaged body, bloated with chemicals and robbed of its vital essence. My mind repeated the mantra: What did they do to you? What did they do to you? What did they do to you?

I was reminded of twenty years earlier, right after the transplant. In stark contrast, Debbie was smiling and waving to me through a glass window in the isolation room. Here her life seemed suspended in an unresolved void. We stood there for about fifteen minutes until the nurse came in and told us it would be good if we left and came back later. We all said our farewells. I kissed my sister on the cheek and whispered, "I love you."

We left the ICU and headed downstairs. It was time for Carolyn and me to head back home. We were numb from seeing Debbie, our senses on override. We said good-bye to my parents. It wasn't easy to leave them. My mother seemed to have her director's hat on though. I could see in her eyes that she was going to do all that she could to make sure that Debbie was comfortable and get the best that the hospital had to give. Somewhere she had found the strength to cope with the situation at hand. I could see more trepidation on my father's face. I could see his mind trying to determine what lie ahead.

We said good-bye to them with smiles and words of hope willed from some inner well of optimism. I wanted to leave my parents feeling that there was hope. At the same time, I was also trying to convince myself that the bad feeling churning in the pit of my stomach was an aberration.

Carolyn and I took a taxi back to the hotel. We had checked out earlier and loaded our bags in the trunk of the car, so that when we returned from the hospital, we could get on the road. We were very anxious to leave Baltimore. Frankly, the last two days left me unsettled and severely shaken, leaving my attempts at a positive attitude badly bruised and depleted.

We left that day, expecting to see my parents and Debbie back at home in a few weeks. I felt that it would probably be closer to three weeks than two as the doctor had said. But I didn't know that the morning before the surgery was the last time that I was to see my sister whole again. And I didn't know it was going to take four months for Debbie to come home.

21

❖ ❖ ❖ ❖

"Dad, are you still outside?" Josh asked, carrying several packages.

"Hi, Josh. I didn't hear you come in."

"Have you been in the backyard all day, Dad?"

"Yeah, I guess I have. Where's your mom?"

"She's right behind me."

"Larry, Josh, what do you guys want for dinner?" Carolyn asked, rushing through the door.

As it turned out, by the time Carolyn had finished her shopping, Joshua was ready to come home from Matt's house. She was able to pick Josh up on her way home. Josh satisfied his yen for hanging out, and Carolyn had accomplished everything she set out to do and then some.

Their sudden return brought a welcome pause to the images replaying in my mind.

"It's 6: 00. Is anyone hungry?" she asked.

"I'm not hungry yet. I had some macaroni and cheese at Matt's house."

"Well, I have nothing in the house, so if you guys want to have dinner you better decide right now. I don't want to hear about it later," Carolyn warned us with half a smile.

"Why don't we bring in some Italian food from Mario's?" I suggested.

"Is that okay with you, Josh?" Carolyn asked.

"I guess so. What can I get?"

"Anything you want. They have pizza, ravioli, garlic bread...." She started going down the menu.

"Whatever you order, Mom, is all right with me."

"Who are you kidding?" I said smiling, "You're the pickiest eater on the planet. Later we'll hear that you're hungry, dinner was horrible, and there's nothing to eat.

"I will not, Dad."

"Larry, what do you want?"

"I'll eat anything you order."

"Ha, that's a joke," Josh said.

"Who are you kidding? You're worse than he is." Carolyn burst in almost simultaneously.

"I am not," I said.

"Yes, you are, Dad," Josh said.

We all started laughing.

"Okay. Why don't we get some ravioli for Josh? You and I can split chicken parmigiana and some eggplant." Carolyn took charge.

"Does that sounds good? Is that okay with you, Josh?" she asked.

"Yeah, it's fine."

"I'll order while you go upstairs and clean your room," Carolyn said to Josh as they started back into the house.

"Do I have to, Mom?" He asked.

The three of us have such a good time. It seems like we've always been together. It's like life before them was another era, another lifetime.

They left me outside with a smile on my face, allowing me to momentarily forget about Debbie's misery. Staring out into the yard, I noticed that the Japanese maple tree we planted this past spring is already starting to shed its leaves. The summer in all its shimmering brilliance will soon give way to fall's radiant colors. The pale of winter will soon subdue nature's hue. For now, though, the vibrant tones of September are on full display delighting the senses.

But every thought of September's glow wanes as the memory of Debbie's travail continues to race across my mind. Things went from bad to worse—and worse still. An unbelievable nightmare continued to unravel my sister's life one step at a time. It was as if everything she had built during her life was being taken away.

Debbie needed three additional surgeries. Her second operation two weeks later was done to reinforce the first surgery with additional bone grafts. Several weeks after that, she needed surgery to swab the original surgical site because an infection threatened everything that had been done to that point. The fourth and final surgery was done because her wound was not closing properly. The surgical area kept on getting infected and threatened her bone grafts. With each ensuing cut of the surgeon's knife, another piece of my sister's psyche lay bare.

My parents stayed with Debbie the entire time she was in the hospital in Baltimore. They lived in the hotel and spent every single day by Debbie's bedside. From early morning till late at night, they watched over her. They endured every surgery, every fever, and every painful scream that my sister had to weather. Their child was caught in the grip of uncertainty. Everyday yielded questions with unsure consequences. There were days that the doctors felt they would have to start all over again. There were days that my sister's spirits were so low and her anguish so great, that she wanted it all to end.

The doctors were also constantly checking whether the cancer had come back. While none of the ceaseless CAT scans and bone scans came back positive, my father always had the hunch that the doctors acted strangely after the test results came back normal. He sensed that they suspected something wasn't quite right–perhaps an undetected cancer somewhere. We all felt that was my father's propensity for assuming the worst. We told him to accept the good results and not to read anything into it. He remained leery nonetheless.

Carolyn, Josh, and I visited Baltimore several times to try to bolster everyone's morale. Instead, we always left feeling over-whelmed, helpless, and powerless to change what my parents and Debbie were going through. We could only sense the chains that bound them together, drowning in a storm of darkness.

We'd go to the hospital with smiles and gifts and news of home. We hoped to find Debbie receptive to our well wishes, but we quickly became subdued. Her room was cold and dreary. The shades were drawn, the sunlight seemingly exiled. The only light came from the muted TV. It was as if night had permanently de-scended upon my sister and my parents in room 212D.

Debbie's suffering hung in the air like a shadowy presence. I can't forget how it bore through my chest, making each breath difficult. I was crestfallen at my sister's anguish. Every attempt to break free and brighten the moments, briefly sparked and dis-solved like a fading flare hopelessly fighting against a blackened sky.

My parents were always happy to see us and tried to rally

hope and the semblance of optimism, but our quick visit couldn't release them from the undertow that was pulling them in.

After five surgeries and three months later, Debbie was stable enough to come back to New York. But she wasn't coming home yet. She still had to learn how to use her legs again. It turned out that she lost more movement in her feet than expected. Her capacity to walk was going to be severely limited, yet there was hope that she would be able to stand and walk with the aid of canes. Her life uncertain and broken, she spent the winter months cloistered in the hollow of a dark and desolate void. We hoped that with springtime's call, the veil of pain would be lifted.

Debbie was transferred to a rehabilitation hospital in Glen Cove, Long Island. It was a combination hospital and physical/occupational rehabilitation center. In addition to physical therapy, Debbie still needed to undergo constant testing to make sure that the cancer hadn't come back and that an infection hadn't developed at the surgical site.

Debbie was having a very difficult time with the prospect of going from one facility to another. After three months away from home, she didn't want anything to do with another institution. She wanted to go home. She wanted to see her family and friends and be warmly and lovingly greeted by her dog and cat that she considered her family.

Not all of Debbie's problems and heartbreaks were medical. In her absence, Carolyn and I took care of her dog and cat. Three weeks after she left for Baltimore and her surgical odyssey began, her dog, Samantha, suddenly got ill. One day she was running around in the backyard with Josh, Molly, and me and then the next day, she couldn't move. She wouldn't eat or walk. I carried her into the car and took her to the vet where her fate was announced. She had about a week to live. She had cancer and heart failure. The vet said the merciful thing to do was to put the dog to sleep. Sam was only eleven years old.

How in the world was I going to tell Debbie? Sam was a member of her family. Debbie had Sam for over ten years. My sister inherited from my mother the knack of always finding an animal in need of a home. Like Rusty, the cat, and Rudy, the donkey-eared German shepherd, Sam was the latest member in my family's tradition of giving a wayward animal a home.

While coming home from work one day, Debbie found Samantha wandering in the front yard. The dog was alone, without identification, looking undernourished and abused. When no one claimed Sam, Debbie adopted and nursed her back to health. Sam joined another of Debbie's refugee take-ins, Chelsea, a stray cat. They both lived together with Debbie in the house she rented in Babylon.

While she was in Baltimore, we agonized over whether to tell Debbie. How could we? We were all afraid that telling Debbie about Sam, with all that my sister had suffered, would throw her off the edge of sanity and into abject despair. We had hoped to delay telling Debbie about her dog as long as possible so that she could become psychologically stronger. She asked about Sam and Chelsea constantly. With all that Debbie had gone through, one of the things she looked forward to the most was having the companionship of her friend, Sam. Now Sam was gone.

Unfortunately, as soon as she was admitted into the rehabilitation center, she asked the doctor if her dog could visit her in the lobby. He agreed that it would be therapeutic and a good idea.

The time had come to tell Debbie about Sam. Carolyn and I decided we had to tell her. When we arrived at the rehab center around 3:00, Debbie had just finished her afternoon therapy session. She was pretty upbeat, and I hesitated telling her. Then she asked when we were going to bring the dog. The timing was apparently inevitable.

The words came out of my mouth; but once they did, I wished them back. Debbie cried inconsolably. It became the psychological straw that broke my sister's back. Debbie's heart was broken and her attempts at rehabilitation suffered a dramatic setback. A shroud of sorrow enveloped her.

Day after day, her ceaseless struggle continued. Debbie still couldn't walk and had to painstakingly learn how to transfer into a chair or a bed. She grappled with learning how to stand. Her success was very limited. She was capable of getting from her bed to a wheelchair and was eventually able to lift herself up onto parallel bars.

While she was in the rehab center, my parents' home was outfitted to make it wheelchair accessible. After a six-week stay, it was time for Debbie to come home. We were all very excited. We made welcome home banners, and Carolyn took Joshua out of school early so that they could hang up all the get well cards she received. We all hoped that coming home would boost Debbie's frame of mind.

It took two hours to get Debbie out of the rehab center. The doctors delayed her release because they, too, had some vague suspicion that something wasn't quite right even though all the tests came back fine. When we finally got the go ahead, we hightailed it out of there as fast as we could fearing that they would change their minds. Debbie was very quiet on the ride home. I think she was quite nervous and apprehensive. She had been away for five months during which time she had lost so much. Physically savaged, mentally despondent, her independence gone, she now was left to try to pick up the pieces, but how?

When we got to my parents' home, Debbie gave a half-hearted smile to the welcome home decorations. She was temporarily exuberant to see her cat again, but her spirits dropped almost instantly as she realized that her dog wasn't there to meet her. She was exhausted from the trip home and after a quick lunch decided to get into bed and take a nap.

22

❖ ❖ ❖ ❖

"Molly, what do you want, girl? What's the matter?"

Molly jumped up with her front paws onto my lap.

"What's the matter? Oh you want some attention, don't you? You're such a good friend, Molly."

Next to their major league appetites, golden retrievers crave attention more than anything else. They give you all their love and affection, nothing held back, but they want all of yours in return. A pat on the head and a few nice words in a high-pitched voice are not sufficient. Nothing short of your undivided devotion will do. I happily give Molly mine.

Carolyn went to pick up the take-out food we had ordered for dinner. Josh decided to go for a ride with her. The restaurant was next to a small toy store and he wanted to get a new football for us to toss around.

Ever since Josh was small, we've enjoyed designing pass routes and throwing a football around in the fall. We huddle up, call a play, Josh runs out, and dives for the pass. Molly, nipping at his heels, tries to take the ball away from him. When she's successful, she runs away enticing us to chase her and taunting us to pry the ball from her bite.

On some Sunday afternoons, Debbie would come by and join us. We'd show Josh some of the plays we used as kids. For Debbie, it brought back the football prowess she first discovered playing ball with me and my friends on the playgrounds of the past.

As the sun sinks below the rooftop, and the shadows grow longer, visions of those happier times, of Debbie and Josh and me, rapidly begin to fade away. I am quickly brought back to the events of this past year. The air that earlier had warmed me now feels chilly. Molly has gone off scouting the corner of the yard. I feel alone.

I can't imagine how isolated Debbie must have felt. Though my mom was by her side constantly, my sister owned her pain. She always reminded us that we could never understand exactly what she was going through everyday. Indeed she was right. As she mourned her losses, all we could do was sympathize. Yet, all our compassion and concern was never enough to reach across the physical boundary to understand, to feel, and to experience what she had been going through and what she continued to face. It was very frustrating to stand by and watch–unable to supply what was needed to take the pain and sadness away.

Debbie was supposed to continue her physical rehabilitation as an outpatient. She used every possible tactic to delay going back. I think she felt that she had gone through enough and wanted to rest. No more, she must have said to herself. Let me just rest here for awhile without any other complications. The fact was, the longer she waited to continue her rehab, the harder it would become. And the potential to make significant gains meant that she had to get going.

Everything was beginning to take its toll on my parents and on my mom in particular. As before, immediately following the transplant, my mother and sister were joined together. My mom sustained Debbie's every emotional trauma. Sometimes, though, Debbie's dependence made things difficult. Debbie wouldn't let my mother go out even if Carolyn or I went over to be with her.

We all became concerned that Debbie was not making any progress and soon she would become too dependent on my mom. While Debbie talked about gaining her independence again, she was conflicted about it. She wanted it, but she also needed and wanted to be cared for by my mother.

We all gave Debbie sympathy, yet my father, Carolyn, and I felt she had to start making some progress. Besides our compassion, we felt it was our role to be positive and encouraging. While sometimes we commiserated with her, at other times, we felt it important to move her from self-absorption to rejoining the world. At times, that led to friction. She didn't always appreciate our efforts; I think at those times she preferred us to empathize with her suffering. Often, it was hard to balance the effort to persuade and motivate her with our offerings of sympathy.

After weeks of refusing to go on a bus to the rehabilitation center by herself, Debbie gave in and consented to go; but not until my mom agreed to follow behind the bus in her car. Once she started, though, she continued. Her strides were slow; but one day her hard work finally paid off. Debbie walked five feet holding onto parallel bars. She was beginning to make progress. A glimmer of light along with a trace of a smile sanctified the moment.

Debbie was never pain free. Some days were better than others, but everyday she suffered from a throbbing pain that never abated. Soon after she started physical therapy as an outpatient, she began to complain that her pain was increasing. We all thought it was a result of the physical work she was doing in rehab. She wasn't so convinced.

To help Debbie get back into the swing of things, my parents would pack her wheelchair in the trunk and take her for rides in the car. Josh and I took her to the movies once and a few times we all went out to a restaurant. We tried to engage her to participate in as many things as possible to regain a sense of doing things and we tried to set up a routine. For the most part, our efforts failed. We tried to find a norm, but things were not normal.

One June afternoon, I received a call from my father. They had taken a ride to enjoy the springtime weather. On their way out to eastern Long Island, Debbie became ill. She was having a very difficult time breathing, so my parents rushed to the emergency room of Stony Brook Hospital.

My father asked me if Carolyn and I would meet them there. We promptly made arrangements with our next-door neighbor to look after Joshua and off we went. What now, we wondered?

When we arrived at the hospital, we met my parents in the waiting room. The doctors had just left. They told my parents that Debbie had fluid on the lungs and that she should stay in the hospital until they could determine what was causing it.

When we went in to see Debbie in the emergency room, she was scared. She couldn't breathe and felt that something was very wrong.

Though afraid and wanting to go back home, she had no choice but to be admitted into the hospital. The end result was that the doctors did a surgical biopsy of her lung. Another procedure, more discomfort, and more uncertainty. They also relieved the fluid around the lungs that had made it difficult for Debbie to breathe. She felt better and came home.

As in the past, we waited for the telephone call with hope, yet we had all become very leery waiting for doctors' phone calls. Several days went by and some of the results came in. Debbie had cancer in her lungs. The news was devastating. What was worse is that they suspected this wasn't the primary sight. She was readmitted into the hospital to have a CAT scan and a bone scan.

The news was not good. Cancer had redeveloped in her sacrum, the site of the original cancer. More test results showed more cancer. She had probable cancer of the diaphragm and the pericardium. The news was assaulting. There was nowhere to hide, no solace to be found.

The unthinkable was now reality. All of the surgeries, all the emotional and physical pain Debbie endured, weren't going to save her. All the hoping that her struggle would give her a chance to go on, couldn't change the outcome. "What did I do wrong?" she asked. "I'm not a bad person. Why did this happen to me?" None of us could answer why this happened to her. Her question was also our question and will forever echo in our hearts.

My father confided in me that when my sister was desperately ill with her kidney disease, he would cry in the basement of his store hiding behind the stock shelves so no one would see him. He said, "I felt so helpless then, there was so little I could do to change the situation. Now it's happening all over again."

My heart cried for my parents. To see the pain that they were enduring and know that there was nothing I could really do to alleviate their sorrow was almost unbearable. Nothing can quench the flame of despair that accompanies knowing your child is going to die. The hopelessness I felt made me numb. I felt like I was losing all three of them.

We were hoping that that the surgeries in Baltimore would lead to a rebirth much as the transplant had been a chance to begin life anew. The gamble didn't work. Rather than being the beginning of a new life, the surgeries marked the beginning of the end of life.

When we met with the doctors in the hospital, they offered more surgery and chemotherapy. The odds that the surgery and chemotherapy would work was less than five percent. If she were lucky enough to be in this category, however, she wouldn't be cancer free for more than six months because there was nearly a hundred percent chance that it would come back. With all that she had been through, the thought of more surgery ravaging her body, and for what end, was not appealing.

After the doctors left, Debbie asked all of us what we thought. We helped her explore her limited options. In the end, Debbie decided that she would go home. She had enough of the cutting and enough of the poking and prodding. With courage, she had fought the battle that cancer made her fight. She went to the best hospitals, she had the top surgeon, and now she had had enough.

The transplant that had given her new hope and twenty-two additional years of life was also the possible origin of the cancer that had ravaged her body in the end. It was surmised that the drugs that had prevented her body from rejecting the kidney also caused the cancer. There were two possible reasons. Either the prolonged use of these powerful drugs allowed a cancer to develop, or her immune system was too suppressed to allow her body to fight the cancer once it took root.

Before we left the hospital, I found the doctor in the hallway and asked him the question we were all afraid to ask. How long did Debbie have to live? He said six months.

23

❖ ❖ ❖ ❖

My sister didn't live for six more months. She spent the last month of her life living in the house where she grew up. Our family journeyed with her as far as we could until the drugs she was taking to ease her enormous pain made coherent conversation futile. There was one thing that she kept saying over and over again. She kept on telling us the importance of sharing life with others. I am not sure if she was regretting that she didn't share her life enough or if she was coming to terms with some greater reality–a reality that resides on the threshold between life and death–a place where simple truths are revealed to the soul.

There was also a host of friends that came by to visit. One by one, she said good-bye to new friends, old friends, and childhood friends. She lay there reminiscing with some, consoling others, and closing chapters as she went along.

My mother, father, Carolyn, Josh, and I, each in our own way, tried to find a way to say good-bye.

A week before she died, Debbie and I had our last lucid conversation.

"Larry, I'm going to die soon," she said.

"I know, Debbie," I said, resigned.

"I know I didn't always show it, but I want you to know how much I appreciate that you gave me your kidney. It gave me twenty-two years of life I wouldn't have had."

"I know, Deb," I said, though I was embarrassed to accept her thanks. Those were the words that I wanted to hear all of our adult lives and now they had such a hollow ring.

She went on determined to share her feelings with me.

"I was able to accomplish a lot of things. Maybe it didn't always appear that I was happy, but I mostly was. Maybe I didn't love myself as often as I should have, and at times I probably judged myself too harshly. But, I had a good life," she said with resolve. "I had a family that loved and supported me in everything I ever did. You don't know how important that was to me. I had good friends and I was a good friend. I tried to be a good and decent person."

Then suddenly she paused. She pressed her lips together and a tear fell from the corner of her eye. I started to comfort her. She braved her emotions and continued.

"My only regret is I won't be here for Joshua as he grows up. I won't get to see the person he is going to become." She paused again; she was now openly weeping. Barely able to speak, she softly cried, "Please Larry, all I ask is that you don't forget me, don't let Joshua forget me."

I held my sister tightly, and my heart felt as though it was ripping apart.

"We won't ever forget you Debbie. We will always miss you. You've always been a good sister to me. I love you, Debbie. I always have and I always will. I'll never forget all the laughs and smiles we shared."

Now she held me away from her at arms length. Looking directly into my eyes she said, "I love you, too."

I grabbed a few tissues, and we both wiped our eyes and composed ourselves.

"Please look after Mom and Dad. This isn't going to be easy for them, but it will get better. Tell them after awhile it will get better. They have to move on," she said, some of her old psychologist wisdom surfacing.

"Don't worry about Mom and Dad. I'll be there for them," I said.

"I know. I'm getting a little tired, and the pain is starting to come back. I should take some more pain killer and then sleep a little."

"Okay, Debbie. I'll call Mom in. She'll give you a shot of painkiller and I'll see you in a little while."

Debbie was right, of course; it didn't always appear that she was happy. I always thought that my sister had a hard life. She spent her teenage years enduring kidney disease. She never married, never had children, went from job to job, and often seemed sad or troubled. But ultimately, I realized that she had lived her life with courage and dignity and here at death's doorway, she appraised her journey. As God in Genesis proclaims his creation as good, so my sister proclaimed her creation, her life, as good. In the end, she seemed at peace with what her life was all about. She didn't have to look back and think that she had left things undone. She felt satisfied that she accomplished, created, lived, loved, was loved, and shared herself with others.

As Debbie expressed her satisfaction, each moment of the last twenty-two years became more precious. I understood more than ever before what it meant to have given her my kidney. As she gazed from a vantage point I couldn't climb to, she shared her contentment; and when she did, I knew fully what it meant to be a kidney donor.

That was our last real conversation. On the morning of August 13th, my mother called me to come over right away. She didn't think that Debbie would last much longer. When I arrived at my parents' home, Debbie was already gone.

Part Four:
Sunset
Same Day
September 1, 1996

❖ ❖ ❖ ❖

24

❖ ❖ ❖ ❖

The pleasure of the morning sunrise in all its dazzling splendor is now spent. The blazing radiance of the afternoon sun is now completely consumed. Twilight, which gleamed in hues of vivid coral and auburn and indigo, has also found its way home. The sun that lit my way down memory's path is now swallowed by different shades of gray and black.

Death carried my sister away from us. For my parents, it is a blow that will never completely heal. Time soothes the immediacy of emotion, but it never washes it away. It remains with us and comes to our attention—often when we least expect it. It can happen when we hear a song, or see a sunrise, hear the wind howl a name, or even as we sit in the backyard on a sunny day. It can come on at any moment and it is as real as if it was yesterday. For my parents, the wound cuts deep beyond the flesh. The strength and perseverance they willed during Debbie's battle with cancer now must see them through the difficult days ahead.

For me, I am still learning new lessons. I still carry the scar on my body like a war wound as a reminder. Yet, I know that a scar represents both a wound and a healing. Sometimes a wound cuts so deep that it takes a lifetime to heal. The 12-inch scar that coils around the right side of my body runs through me like the lifeline in the palm of my hand.

I shared childhood memories with Debbie that were like secret codes. A word or a gesture that had significance only for the two of us could send us into a fit of uncontrollable laughter. It is an unspoken bond that is triggered by some unexplainable mechanism that can happen just between siblings. Sadly, I miss dearly sharing the memory of those wondrous times with Debbie. Fortunately, I can still smile gently when I think of them. Yet it doesn't seem right that she's not here. I wonder: Where is she?

When someone who is an integral part of our life leaves, a shift in the world takes place. The balance of things comes undone. No one can ever take the place of someone else. The person who is gone takes a piece of the drama with them. Life changes; its equation undergoes a metamorphosis. Relationships recast themselves. So it has been for my family. My parents and I are still an essential part of each other's lives. We share past memories and future dreams. We still lovingly share the joy of being involved in life's milestones. Yet each of us in our own way is left to feel how we were enriched by my sister's life and diminished by her death.

"Dad, it's time for dinner," Josh yelled as he and Carolyn came through the door.

"Okay, Josh. I'll be right there."

But I just sit here unable to move, tears streaming down my cheek. Just like this morning in the shower, I hold my trembling hands to my face and weep. My lips, unable to sustain a sound, mouth "I miss you, Debbie." And at the same time, my heart aches knowing I will miss her every day for the rest of my life.

"Dad, come on. Mom has it on the table and I'm hungry."

"Okay, Josh," I say in a whisper.

Molly comes over to see why I seem so troubled. She looks up to me with concerned eyes, as if to say, "Don't cry. It will be all right." I fumble for a crumpled tissue lodged in the corner of my pocket and start to compose myself.

"Dad, we're waiting."

I've got to go now. My family calls me, life calls me, and it holds me to its bargain. It breathes through me. It beckons to me. Life sighs live, love, share, and create. As it does, I hear it beating in my chest.

"Larry, come in now. You've been outside all day. It's time to come in and eat dinner," Carolyn called out the kitchen window.

"Okay, I'm coming now. I'm finished."

"Molly, come girl, let's go inside."

She runs to the door, wagging her tail. I follow in her foot-steps. I turn to look back and think that time goes by too fast–day after day, week by week, month by month, year after year, until a whole lifetime is done, come and gone almost in an instant. Our moments are strung together, a tapestry of experiences that adorn our soul's eternal heart. Our star rises, glistening light across the river of life, caressing its sweet essence. Then it sets, saying fare-well, and contemplating its sojourn.

The things that happen to us happen for a reason. We may not always know why things occur to us at the time they do, but somewhere the answer lies deep within the fabric of our spirit. At times, we yearn for understanding. At other times, we feel satiated. We endure moments of anxiety, questioning our uncertain future, but we also experience flashes of absolute lucidity when we can see from one end of the universe to the other and hold its entirety within our very being.

The sum of our lives is more than folly. Our lives point us to a greater reality that, when taken as a whole, tells us how far we've reached and how much further we have to go.

We are courageous warriors and wayward travelers. We are bold and brave, yet we are humbled and frightened. We seek to better ourselves, yet we wallow in self-pity. We are all these things hurling through space, but we are more. We are in the process of achieving and creating. We are evolving toward our destiny to be more than we were yesterday. Our collective lives are unfolding to reveal ourselves as divine creatures created in a divine image. We are learning that what we forsake as mundane is really sacred.

Every breath is sacred. Life is sacred.

I look up into the sky and say goodnight. My day's reflection feels witnessed by a power greater than me. Goodnight, God. Watch over us. Watch over all of us.

"Dad, we can't wait any longer. We're eating."

"Don't start without me. I'm starved."

Epilogue

Five Months Later:

Midnight on January 31, 1997

Our house is quiet now. A gentle breeze taps at the window. Sleep eludes me. Carolyn rests effortlessly beside me. She has always been a better sleeper. I walk down the darkened hall and into the living room. I'm drawn to the bay window, which overlooks our well-kept suburban lawn. Sitting down at the edge of the hassock, I stare into the night. Molly comes over to me and sits down as if in the front row waiting for the show to begin. Both of us have our faces close to the window; our breath condenses on the glass. Harmless large white flakes start to fall. The breeze softly swirls them around, drifting surrealistically to the ground. The snow that had been predicted earlier has finally arrived. This is winter's first snowfall.

With the realization that the years are passing by too quickly, I've come to look forward to the first snow. Memories resurface. There is a recounting of childhood snow scenes, forever etched in my mind of my mom, dad, and sister. Thoughts of snowballs and snowmen and ice castles brighten my mind.

With a smile on my face, I think of tomorrow morning–with the snow glistening two to three inches thick on the tree branches in a soft sunlight. Tomorrow Josh will put on his snow pants and the four of us will smile and laugh as we make snowballs, and snowmen, and ice castles–and memories.

Softly, barely audible, I ask, "Who am I?" Hopeful and attentive, I search the night for a response. There is none, yet I don't feel alone. I don't feel insignificant. Then I ask why am I here. I am forty-five years old, more than half my years vanished. Everything that has happened to me has led me to this moment.

My sister is gone now and I am the keeper of the memories we shared. I wonder what life would have been like had Debbie not had a rare kidney disease and I hadn't given her my kidney twenty-three years ago today. How different would our lives have been–Debbie's, my parents', and mine? But our drama unfolded the way it did for a reason, each of us playing a different role and each of us affecting the other and influencing the lens through which we see the world.

The snow now driving hard against the window momentarily interrupts my thought. I look at Molly peering out over winter's work. But suddenly my mind shifts. Life's mirror struggles to reflect a buried truth, a message, twisted in an odd shape, pulling and stubbornly tugging at my heart. Suddenly there's a wound striving to surface, looking for peace–a deep hurt immersed in dark guilt. There, openly exposed, my hurt, my guilt, and my disappointment after the transplant. It seems so hollow, so unseemly.

Why does it surface now? Why now, when I mourn for my sister, when I grieve for the heartache of my parents? Can it be that only now my disappointment with Debbie and my parents, rising from the depth, can be discharged? I allow its memory of loneliness and isolation to rush over me and recall after the kidney transplant how I was saddened because I felt wounded, and confused. I didn't feel acknowledged for what I had done. But these feelings were at odds with what I required of myself. I expected to be the perfect hero. I expected this to be the perfect gift given in the perfect way–a gift that is given out of love with no special response or acclaim necessary. I found it hard to accept that part of me needed to be acknowledged. I denied it. I drove that impulse deep inside my psyche out of shame and guilt because I felt it diminished the spirit in which I gave Debbie my kidney.

Now though, these emotions strike my heart like an arrow piecing hardened armor. Could it be that I couldn't accept my deepest thoughts and feelings? Could it be that I needed to feel and know that it was okay for me to want to be acknowledged for donating my kidney to Debbie? Could it be that I needed to see that I didn't have to be perfect? Could it be that simple? I gaze into my heart and in an instant know it to be true.

Only the briefest of moments pass but there dwelling in the center of my being comes the understanding that my parents and Debbie didn't need to be perfect either.

Then suddenly, the light that led my way through my memory, down through my emotions, is gone, but in its wake, the ache that lodged itself in the vein of my spirit, is soothed.

I had donated my kidney to my sister out of love. In the purest sense it was a gift from my heart that said I love you. Often, however, the decisions we make are layered with a variety of motivations. As I discovered, in part, I had also donated my kidney to my sister wanting to receive love as well. It was a gift that said I need love, too. Because love is so powerful, it is often expressed in awkward and imperfect ways.

The street light silhouettes the snow now slowly descending, floating rhythmically to an unknown meter. Each flake is seemingly distinct from the other. I wonder: Does everyone who has ever lived yearn for the same thing–wanting wholeness, wanting to create something, looking to be noticed, seeking to love, and be loved?

It's been five months since my sister's death and I am still left wondering about her life. Was she able to come to terms with the transplant saga? Did her experience gnaw at her from somewhere beyond the conscience mind? Did she ever come to terms with the part I played?

While sorting through her things, I came across several journals. One journal was an account of her life in the late 1980's that left me wondering if she was really happy with her life. It was a time marked with melancholy and she was feeling very lonely. In one six-month period, when she was about thirty-one, she wrote several times about suicide. She mused about how to arrange it all.

At first, when I read what she wrote, I cried. Why didn't I know how she felt? Then I became angry. How could she think like that? What would make her feel that way? How ironic, with all we went through. How could she have considered taking her own life, knowing the mental and emotional distress that my parents suffered? What could she have possibly thought of the physical and emotional sacrifice I endured for her?

But the more I thought about it, the more I tossed it around in my mind, I began to see things differently. A second look revealed another truth. At the very moment of deep despair, facing her darkest thoughts, when life seemed too much to bare, she emerges from the depth of heartache and unequivocally rejects death as a solution. Rather, she chooses to rise from the ash of hopelessness to reaffirm her faith in life and renews its contract.

Who can fathom someone else's struggle and drama? Who can fully know the gifts and tasks with which someone is born? Who can tell the ultimate purpose of their life, and whether they have succeeded? My sister and God stand as witness and arbiter of her drama. Those that she left behind are left to assess the impact she had on their life.

After Debbie died, countless friends called and visited. Some spoke to my parents and some to Carolyn and me.

I specifically remember Debbie's friend, Sally, saying in a soft reflective voice, "Thank you for giving Debbie your kidney. If you didn't, she wouldn't have been there for me when I was going through my most desperate moment. I was so overwhelmed with everything that was going wrong in my life. Debbie was there for me to talk to, to cry to, and to just keep me company. I can't tell you what that meant to me. She was so generous to me. To know that someone cared enough to listen. I'm going to miss Debbie terribly. She was very special."

Ultimately, I realize a simple truth. I was blessed to be able to give my kidney to my sister. The outpouring of love and tears after my sister's death was a tribute to the way in which she lived. Her journey had significant meaning to those who came in contact with her. It is an eloquent reminder how one life affects so many others.

The second journal I found was written in 1975, a year after the transplant operation. In it was a letter to me:

Dear Larry,

This is a letter written especially for you. I want to express in words my feelings of appreciation. You mean so much to me. You have given me a lot of meaningful things. Especially, though, you have showed me the importance and meaning of love. You put your life on the line, risking so much so I could have a chance to live again. You gave me your love and the opportunity for a new life by donating your kidney to me. What more can we expect in life but to have love for one another?

I realize no one really acknowledged what you did for me, including me. I just want to say thank you. Thank you for my new happy and healthy life. Thank you for sharing your life with me. Most important, thank you for being you.

Love,
Debbie

There it was! The thank you I had looked for all these years in a letter that was never sent. So many thoughts went around in my mind. Mostly, I wondered why Debbie never sent the letter to me. Maybe she meant to, maybe she couldn't, maybe she felt it didn't express enough. Maybe the dynamics of sibling rivalry wouldn't allow her to send it. Maybe it wasn't perfect. Maybe it made her feel vulnerable. Whatever it was, I'm glad to have found it, but I am sad that we weren't able to share it together.

An illness, a letter never sent, lessons learned, and the direction of many lives is affected. Among the lessons is the happiness of giving. It's the joy that comes from opening your heart and saying, "I want to share something of myself with you. Please accept it." In essence, when you give a gift, the act of giving generates warmth inside the soul. Gifts come in many packages. Some gifts are as subtle as sharing a smile. Others have a bigger impact, like donating a kidney. But when we give, it enables us to show and feel the love we have for someone else. Being able to express love is the most compelling and dynamic force we can share. Sharing our love connects us to our own souls. It connects us to each other. It connects us to God.

There is a saying: "Whoever preserves a single soul, it is as though they saved a complete world." Somehow this saying seems incomplete because it also has to be said that in helping someone else, we ultimately help ourselves—in essence we save our own world as well. So I recall Dr. Collins' words to me the night before the transplant. He told me that I was fortunate to be able to give my sister this gift. Now more than ever, I have come to realize that not only did giving my kidney to Debbie make a profound difference in her life, it also made all the difference in my life as well.

The snow is now driving hard and the wind gusts wildly, squalling, fiercely scraping the barren tree branches across the side of the house. The cold bites through a small crack in the window. Only moments ago, nature's scene was calming, serene, beautiful. Now it feels unforgiving. How curious is nature's way—both wondrous and afflicting. Our lives, too, are filled with beauty and pain.

I can't say why my sister had to endure the hardship she did. I don't know why any of us do. What I do know is that our lives are forged from the fire of experience. We are molded by it and tempered by it. We are challenged by it. We affect others and they affect us. Our actions have consequences. If we learn from each other and share ourselves, our lives are enriched. Life is then filled with meaning.

There is an ancient story about what happens to us before we are born. It is said that an angel appears before us and shows us a light that enables us to see all things. Everything is explained to us—why we live and why we die, and what our earthly tasks are. There we are bathed in the light of all knowing. Then right before we are born, the angel causes us to forget everything that was just shown to us.

When I hear this story, I always wonder why we have to

forget. The answer is always the same. We forget in order that we may enter the drama and experientially awaken a little bit at a time to the awareness that God's presence is everywhere–within the beauty of a floating snowflake, and even in the hardship we endure.

The snow squalls ebb. Only a few flakes remain, half-heartedly falling, uncertain whether to complete the journey earthbound. A coat of pristine white crystal now blankets the ground. The night is still and even the wind whispers silently. Only the sound of my heart beating invades the quietness. I feel myself resonating from a place within, where I am in accordance with all of nature, a seamless unity with the rest of the world.

So who am I? I am defined and bound by my past, yet limitless as to who I might be now and in the future. While I am husband, father, son, writer, and kidney donor, I cannot be limited. Life compels me to move forward and become more. Its essence flows through me and reminds me to create and renew myself and to be grateful for my experiences. But at the same time it also implores me to look to my own heart and accept myself for who I am.

As the sunrise reminds us of the newness of each day, so, too, life gestures–come, be a part of the mystery I put before you. Enter the tales of beauty, of sadness, of joy, of courage and of...

Molly pokes my hand with her cold nose, wanting to be petted. Looking at me, she wags her tail. I oblige her and say it's time to go to sleep, girl. She follows me down the hall back toward the bedrooms. I stop at Joshua's room. I look in on my son finally sleeping after struggling to stay awake just a moment longer. I walk over to him, unfold the small quilt he has had since his birth and softly cover him. I listen to him gently breathing and then kiss him on the head. Quietly I whisper, "Goodnight, my little boy. I love you."

I turn and walk into my bedroom. Molly goes over to her corner. She puts her head down, closes her eyes, and sighs. I say, "Goodnight, girl. I'll see you in the morning."

I arrange the pillows the way I like them and hop into bed. Carolyn's still sound asleep. I lean over quietly, kiss her cheek, and say, "Goodnight, sweetheart." She wrestles around a bit, pulls the blankets tightly around her shoulders, and says to me, "Goodnight. I love you." I say, "I love you too, sweetie."

I wrap myself in the blankets, feeling safe and warm. I feel myself drifting off to sleep thinking about tomorrow. We'll anxiously bundle ourselves in our winter wear, open the door, and vault ourselves into the untouched snow on the ground. Our footprints will dot winter's landscape, leaving the unblemished snow changed forever by our presence. We will share in the delight of being together, shoveling the snow, and throwing snowballs for Molly to fetch.

I think to myself that we are here for such a short time, but I also know that everything we do matters. I sense that our lives, planted here on the earth, also soar through the heavens. What we do together weaves the very fabric of life. When we support each other and rejoice in each other's lives, we find fulfillment. When we nurture and help each other grow, we discover that we have a chance to appreciate the most precious gift of all: sharing life with the people we love-not only times of happiness and joy but the difficult and desperate moments as well. And then, after sharing our lives, when we leave with our footprint on its landscape, life is forever changed by our presence.

I wrestle with the blankets and Carolyn complains that I am taking all the covers.

"Larry, go to sleep already. Tomorrow is another day."

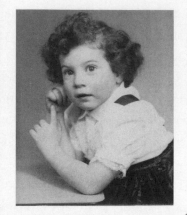

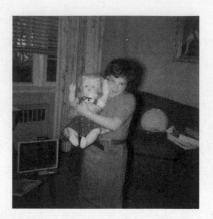

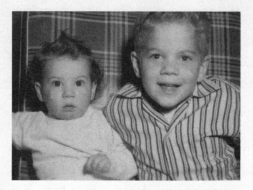

Above left and lower right: Debbie and I spent a day posing for pictures in my grandfather's photography studio in Brooklyn, New York. *Above right*: Debbie is obviously pleased with a new doll. *Middle left*: Debbie and I were allowed to stay up late one evening. *Bottom left*: my mom, Debbie and I around the kitchen table with my dad behind the camera.

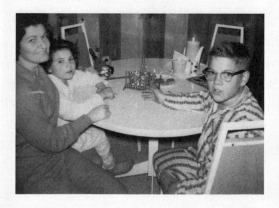

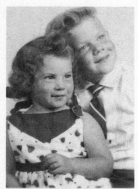

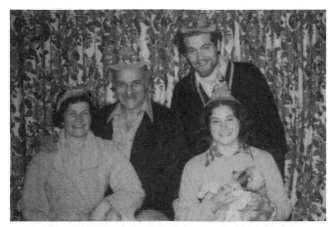

Debbie, my mom, dad and I celebrating Debbie's birthday.

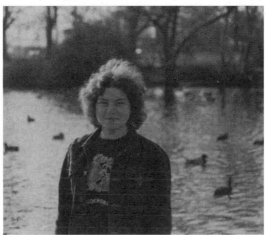

Debbie enjoying the quiet of a nearby pond.

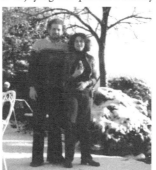

February, 1978, four years after
the transplant.